# Somatic Exercises For Seniors

Reduce Anxiety, Regain Posture With 15-Min Calming Exercise Book

© **COPYRIGHT LUNA LIGHT. ALL RIGHTS RESERVED.**

No part of this book may be reproduced, distributed, or transmitted in any form or by any means, including photocopying, recording, or other electronic or mechanical methods, without the prior written permission of the publisher, except in the case of brief quotations embodied in reviews. Unauthorized reproduction or distribution of this work, or any portion of it, may result in civil and criminal penalties as prosecuted under Sections 107 and 108 of the 1976 United States Copyright Act and any copyright laws in the country of the violator.

**DISCLAIMER**

This book is intended to provide readers with general information about yoga exercises and routines. The content provided is not a substitute for professional medical advice, diagnosis, or treatment. Engaging in any exercise program carries the risk of injury. While the author and publisher have made every effort to ensure the safety of the exercises and routines described in this book, they cannot guarantee that they are appropriate for every individual. Always seek the advice of a qualified healthcare provider with any questions you may have regarding a medical condition or physical exercise regimen if you are unsure. If you experience pain, dizziness, discomfort, or any other symptoms while performing any of the exercises described in this book, stop immediately and consider seeking medical attention. By voluntarily participating in any of the exercises shown in this publication, you accept the risk of any potential injury.

## YOUR FREE GIFTS

Congrats! Your book comes with 3 bonus e-books. All you have to do is go to wallpilates.org to download them.

# Contents

## YOUR FREE VIDEOS

Your purchase of this book comes with over 101 videos to help you visualize the somatic movements in this book.

Just write an email to **wallpilates2@gmail.com** with the subject line: **somatic videos** and we'll send it to you promptly.

# **Introduction**

How did I end up like this?

It was a question that 72-year-old Jane asked herself often. She had resigned herself to shuffling through her days burdened by the weight of chronic pain. Each step felt like trudging through quicksand; her back ached with every movement, and even the simplest tasks became herculean feats.

As she watched the world around her bustle with life, Jane couldn't help but feel like a spectator in her own existence. The once vibrant, energetic woman was now enveloped in a cocoon of discomfort, pain, and tension.

Maybe you feel a bit like Jane.

You're not alone.

When we reach the age of 60, everything starts to hurt: the back, shoulders, hamstrings, and even the calf muscles. Yet, we don't really understand why. We've been conditioned to accept it as a consequence of getting older. So, people tell us that we need to start slowing down.

Sometimes, our bodies end up with trapped tension at a younger age.

Yet, you were created to move—and to keep moving—despite the advancing years. Forcing ourselves to stop moving is the worst thing we can do.

The problem is not that you're getting old. It's that you have developed sensory motor amnesia.

It's a term that few people are familiar with, yet it affects the vast majority of us. It causes all those aches and pains that cause so much discomfort, making simply getting through the day feel like climbing Mount Everest.

So, what is sensory motor amnesia?

It is when the brain loses awareness and control over our muscles and movement patterns. It develops over time as a result of poor movement habits, bad posture, stress, and emotional trauma.

Sensory muscle amnesia is the root cause of chronic muscular tension, pain, and movement restriction.

Somatic movement is the remedy for sensory motor amnesia. It teaches you to regain muscle sensation and control through gentle movement patterns. Once you can regain that sensory control and rid yourself of the amnesia that has been causing your pain, miraculous things start to happen ...

- You're able to walk with confidence

- You can dance like you did 20 years ago

- That chronic lower back pain is gone (not just lessened but completely eliminated!)

- Your level of self-confidence and independence will go through the roof

And all you've done is help your brain remember the proper ways to move, which have been forgotten over the years.

Hi, my name's Luna. I'm a Pilates and yoga instructor with a special affinity for working with people from all walks of life. I'm passionate about helping older folks rid their bodies of pain and live their best lives. I was introduced to somatic exercises about ten years ago when I read a book called *Move Without Pain* by Martha Peterson.[1]

Since then, I've become a somatics convert. I believe that somatics should be taught in every retirement home, every doctor should prescribe it, and every individual should have access to this transformative practice.

While sometimes, there is a physical issue related to bad posture or pain-related movements, my clients often come to me after they have done all the tests (MRI, ultrasound, bloodwork) and can still find nothing wrong with their bodies! This is where we shift to the focus to somatic movements, and start becoming aware of your

---

1    Peterson, M. (2012). *Move Without Pain*. Union Square & Co.

muscles, your focus, and your connection between the mind and body. Even if you do have a physical issues, Somatics can still help in your healing process. It's important for me to say here that I am not a doctor and sometimes there are rare and difficult cases of pain that's unresolved through  movement alone. However, the studies show that most people who live with tension and pain, especially chronic pain, always have a psychological and movement component in their recovery process.

"Perhaps 85 percent of patients with isolated low back pain cannot be given a precise pathoanatomical diagnosis. The association between symptoms and imaging results is weak", according to the New England Journal Of Medicine[2]. This is why its so important to continue to move even if you're in pain. Unless there is a specific, acute sprain or detectable injury, most pain becomes chronic because the brain is misfiring signals. In these cases, we can use Somatics to train your body to feel safe through the power of these movements.

To help you understand why, let's get back to Jane.

Jane turned up at my studio one day, hunched over a walker and obviously in discomfort. I knew immediately that she was a prime candidate for somatics. After some convincing, she decided to give it a try. Little did she know that this decision would mark the beginning of a remarkable journey.

As Jane tentatively engaged in the gentle movements prescribed by somatics, she felt a stirring within her body. Layers of discomfort began to peel away, engaging muscles that had grown accustomed to dormancy.

Slowly but surely, Jane's strides grew more confident, her once-hunched shoulders squared with newfound strength, and the burden that had weighed her down for years began to lift. She was becoming pain-free. Within a few months, Jane's mind became sharper,  and her mood stabilized at a more energetic level.

Now it's your turn.

---

2    Deyo & Weinstein (2001). "Low Back Pain." *New England Journal of Medicine.*

# Essential Knowledge

# **What Is** Somatics?

The word somatic literally means "of or relating to the human body." It is a scientific term that has become popular in different forms of exercise and healing. You may have heard of somatic yoga, somatic therapy, somatic psychology, or somatic dance therapy.

Somatic education was pioneered by an American philosopher and therapist named Thomas Hanna. He was very interested in the mind-body connection and sought to understand how chronic stress, habitual movement patterns, and emotional factors contribute to muscular tension and pain.

Hanna combined neurophysiology and human movement to develop a method for teaching people how to regain control of their muscles and movement patterns, thereby relieving chronic pain and improving overall well-being.

Hanna Somatic Education is based on the premise that chronic muscular tension is often the result of learned patterns of muscular contraction and can be alleviated through awareness and voluntary control of these patterns. Hanna developed a series of gentle, mindful movements called "pandiculations" to help people release chronic tension and restore healthy movement patterns.

These movements are performed slowly and with focused attention to reprogram the neuromuscular system and regain flexibility, coordination, and comfort.

Clinical Somatic Education (CSE) teaches how to release chronic muscle tension and improve posture so you can get out of pain and stop doing damage to your body. Most pain in the body results from habitual standing and movement patterns that have developed over a person's lifetime. As a result of muscle memory, we slip into the same unhealthy patterns of movement hundreds of times daily without even thinking about it.

These patterns are hard to change. We certainly can't do it with conventional exercises like squats and push-ups. Massage, chiropractic, or strength training won't do it, either. Getting rid of the postures, stances, and movement patterns at the root of physical pain can only occur through clinical somatic education (CSE).

CSE teaches you to release chronic muscle contraction systematically. Once you have rid your body of these destructive patterns, you slowly introduce efficient, natural full body movement patterns to promote greater ease of movement and overall well-being.

Proprioceptive exercises are also introduced to improve posture and enhance body awareness, completing the process of retraining the body to move efficiently and without pain.

# **Why** It Works

The key to understanding why somatics is so effective is to realize that pain is a consequence of your body's habitual movement patterns. By learning and applying somatic exercises, you can address the root cause of your pain, gradually and permanently find relief, improve your posture, and calm your mind.

Let's consider the principles that are the foundation of Thomas Hanna's clinical somatic education:

01   **Chronic muscular-skeletal pain, dysfunctional posture and movement, and physical degeneration usually result from learned muscular patterns.** The nervous system controls our muscles. The instructions the nervous system relays to the muscles about standing and moving directly relate to the chronic pain, degeneration, and misalignment you may be experiencing.

Other causes, such as genetic factors, nervous system disease, and diet, may exist. However, once these are eliminated, it is almost certain that your pain is caused by learned habitual motor patterns.

**02  Active Movement is the instrument of positive change.** Passive interventions like massage and chiropractic will only provide temporary relief. Only active movement can form new and better neural pathways.

**03  For real, lasting pain relief, you must address the root cause of the problem.** Many so-called pain treatments only mask the pain by treating the symptoms. Somatics works with your nervous system to correct whole-body movement patterns.

**04  Your body's core is the foundation of whole-body movement.** You should work the core first to build a stable base for all your movement patterns.

**05  The goal of somatics is for you to become self-sufficient rather than dependent.** You will learn to rely on yourself rather than the crutch of a therapist or medication.

# How to Perform
## Somatic Movements

Somatic movements are done consciously, with a strong mind-muscle connection. You should focus on the movement's internal experience rather than the end result or external experience.

This is very different from most forms of exercise. When we do movements like squats or bicep curls, we tend to focus on counting the repetitions until we complete a set. In yoga, we might focus on extending our arms overhead and twisting our torso.

With somatics, you should focus your attention entirely on what you feel and experience as you move. This will help you discover the unique tension patterns deeply embedded in your nervous system.

The main thing is not the quantity or intensity of the movement. Instead, the quality of internal exploration and conscious attention is paramount.

I suggest you practice the lying down somatic movements with your eyes closed. This will remove any visual inputs that may distract your attention and allow you to focus internally.

Some of the exercises will be performed standing on the floor or sitting in a chair. If possible, you should perform these movements in front of a mirror. This allows you to combine your internal sense of correct alignment with what you are looking at in the mirror and gives you a greater awareness of proper posture.

You should perform your somatic movements very slowly, especially at the start. It takes time for your nervous system to embed new pathways. Be patient with yourself, and don't push it. Your goal is to make permanent changes!

I recommend not participating in other exercises or muscle treatment while following your 28-day somatics therapy program. Doing so may actually be counterproductive as it can make your muscles tighter. It may also confuse the nervous system as you attempt to adapt your learned movement patterns.

So, if you have been having deep tissue massage or spinal adjustments, you should pause them during this program. You should also stop doing any intense stretching or strength training.

Putting these practices on hold may be pretty difficult for you. You may look forward to them and reap some immediate relief. However, **I'm asking you to have faith that somatic therapy will provide you with far superior, long-lasting results**. Once your nervous system has been reeducated, you can gradually incorporate your previous exercise habits into your lifestyle.

Practice your somatic movements for a few minutes every day. The daily reinforcement of your neural inputs will slowly but surely bring about the changes your body craves.

# Is Somatics Right for Me?

Somatic training is an accessible form of exercise for everyone. But it is especially beneficial for seniors. Its slow, gentle movements allow you to work within your current physical limitations.

You don't have to be fit or strong to get started. In fact, your current condition doesn't matter. Every exercise can be modified so you can perform it comfortably. Most movements are performed lying down, though those designed to modify your posture are done sitting or standing.

# How It's Different

- Somatic technique exercises focus on addressing the root cause of pain by reprogramming learned muscular patterns, whereas traditional forms of exercise may primarily target symptom relief.

- Somatic exercises are performed consciously with a strong mind-muscle connection, emphasizing internal experience rather than external results, contrasting with the focus on completing sets or achieving specific poses in traditional exercise.

- Somatic movements are performed slowly and with focused attention, allowing for the exploration and release of tension patterns embedded in the nervous system, as opposed to the often faster-paced and externally oriented nature of traditional exercises.

- Somatic education promotes self-sufficiency and empowerment by teaching people to rely on themselves rather than external interventions, in contrast to the potential dependency on therapists or medications in traditional pain treatments.

- Somatic movements prioritize the quality of internal exploration over the quantity or intensity of the movement, fostering gradual and lasting changes in the nervous system, unlike the emphasis on external performance metrics in traditional exercise.

- During a somatics program, it is recommended to avoid other forms of exercise or muscle treatments, as they may interfere with the process of neural reeducation, which differs from traditional approaches that may incorporate a variety of interventions simultaneously.

- Somatic therapy encourages patience and consistency in practice, with the understanding that permanent changes take time to embed in the nervous system, contrasting with the potential for immediate relief and varied exercise routines in traditional approaches.

The 3 somatic reflexes are:

Green light reflex     Red light reflex     Trauma reflex

For more information, please read *Somatics* by Thomas Hanna.[3]

---

3    Hanna, Thomas. (2004). *Somatics: Reawakening the Mind's Control of Movement, Flexibility, and Health.*

And for further information about the theories of functional integration, please read his book, *The Body of Life: Creating New Pathways for Sensory Awareness and Fluid Movement.*[4]

---

4    Hanna, T. (1993). *The Body of Life: Creating New Pathways for Sensory Awareness and Fluid Movement.*

I want to remind you that a free gift comes with your purchase of this book: *the Ultimate Kegels Guide.*

This guide helps you strengthen your core and improve your intimate life. Kegels are often done incorrectly, but these instructions are from Tim Sawyer, a top physical therapist who worked with doctors at Stanford University[5] to develop chronic pain rehabilitation programs.

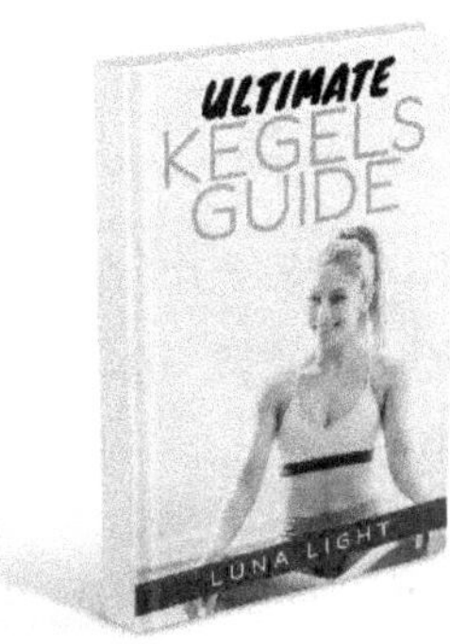

All you have to do is go to wallpilates.org to download it for free. Alternatively, scan the QR code below:

---

5    Dr. Wise and Dr. Anderson *authored A Headache in the Pelvis: A New Understanding and Treatment for Chronic Pelvic Pain Syndromes* (Harmony: 2018) and consulted Tim as the main physical therapist for their treatments.

# **Stretching**
## vs. Pandiculation

Rather than traditional stretching, somatics makes use of a technique called pandiculation. There are three stages of pandiculation:

**01**   Voluntary muscle contraction

**02**   Slow, controlled release of muscle tension

**03**   Total muscle relaxation

Let's practice pandiculation right now. We'll focus on our shoulders, where many people experience tension. Close your eyes and bring your left shoulder up toward your ear. Tighten the muscles slightly.

Now, slowly release the shoulder back down. Allow it to flow gently back to its normal position. Relax that shoulder completely, allowing it to soften and melt down.

Notice the difference between your two shoulders. The one you just pandiculated will feel a lot freer.

Repeat the process with the other shoulder. If you notice tension or jumpiness in the shoulder on the way down, stop and bring it back up to your ear, then very slowly go back down.

Somatics makes use of pandiculation to safely and gently connect with your physical self and relieve chronic pain.

Pandiculation is an example of an active movement pattern. You contract and slowly lengthen the muscles while engaging your brain and nervous system.

Stretching, however, is an example of a passive movement. You passively pull the muscle to extend its length.

Pandiculation has been called "nature's reset button" because it resets the connection between the central and muscular systems. Importantly, unlike stretching, it does this both during muscle contraction and relaxation.

Pandiculation is actually built into us, as it is with all vertebrates. We call it the yawning and stretching, and you probably did it when you got out of bed this morning.

A significant difference between stretching and pandiculation is that stretching works on individual muscles, whereas pandiculation addresses how muscles work together as a functional whole. This allows us to release tension within the muscles far more effectively.

Unlike stretching, pandiculation requires a complete mind-muscle connection. During the second phase–the slow, controlled release–your brain takes back control of the muscle's length and function, and this reeducation of the brain's sensory ability to control the muscle results in permanent changes.

Unlike stretching, pandiculation should never feel painful. Instead, it should feel like a refreshing yawn for the part of the body being worked on.

# How to Turn a Stretch
## into a Pandiculation

Pandiculation is at the very heart of somatics. A pandiculation contracts muscles and then slowly releases them. In contrast, a stretch triggers the stretch reflex, which makes the muscles want to tighten back up. Here are some examples of turning stretches into pandiculations.

To turn a side stretch into a pandiculation, sit alongside a bench or table that is at the same height as your chair. Place your hands on the table (body width) and press into the table. Feel your abdominals contract on the side closest to the table as the other side lengthens. Now use your hand to tap the obliques to really feel the contraction.

Now, very slowly release as you come back to an upright position, lengthening and rotating out of it.

To turn an overhead chest stretch with a bar (or length of dowel) into a pandiculation, stand with a bar in your hands, held wider than shoulder width at arm's length. Now round your shoulders inward, and put a little pressure inward as if you were pushing your hands toward each other. You will feel this through the biceps, chest, and anterior deltoids.

Slowly release and bring the bar up to the chest. This opens and lengthens the chest. Finally, slowly lower the back down to arm's length.

Note: To fully understand pandiculation, please watch this video by my mentor Martha:

https://www.youtube.com/watch?v=Bu47eJ-VNNI&t=211s

If you're reading this in print, search for "Stretching vs. Pandiculation by Essential Somatics."

# **Somatic** Breathing

Breathing is about more than getting oxygen into your body. In fact, the way we breathe often reflects the way we live. Unfortunately, many people have developed a less-than-ideal breathing pattern: they breathe shallowly, only utilizing the upper portion of their lungs, and often hold their breath unconsciously, especially during times of stress or intense concentration.

This restricted breathing limits the amount of oxygen that reaches their cells and perpetuates a cycle of tension and anxiety in both body and mind.

Somatics has the power to revolutionize your breathing. When you pandiculate the muscles of your body's front, back, and sides, you'll relieve excess tension from your breathing muscles.

The inability to breathe correctly is a form of sensory motor amnesia. It often shows up as a locked-down rib cage. When you breathe, the rib cage doesn't move as it should, so less oxygen is taken into the body. This reduces the oxygen uptake to the heart and brain, negatively affecting every body part.

Stress and trauma can also restrict breathing. Somatics teaches you to relax fully and be present with your body. Your stress and trauma will dissipate, allowing you to breathe the way you are meant to.

Here is an exercise that will help you connect with how your rib cage should move as you breathe:

**01**  Stand with your hands on your ribs and breathe naturally. Notice if you feel any movement through your hands.

**02**  If you don't feel movement through the hands, check if your shoulders are rising or only your belly is moving. If so, your locked rib cage is preventing you from breathing correctly.

**03**  Now, take a deep, inward breath, expanding your rib cage on the inhale.

**04**  Exhale slowly.

**05**  Inhale again, and this time, draw your shoulder blades down and back.

**06**  Slowly release, allowing your rib cage to move back to center.

**07**  Do this one more time.

**08**  Place your right hand on your right rib cage, with the left arm at your side.

**09**  Breathe in.

**10**    As you exhale, feel your ribs lean to the right side. You will feel a slight stitch sensation on that side.

**11**    Inhale.

**12**    Repeat on the other side.

This exercise allows you to identify the movement patterns you've developed that may impede your breathing. Stress or tension may be causing you to lock up your rib cage, tense your back muscles, or lean to one side when you breathe. All of these things will restrict your breathing.

The somatics exercises in Section II of this book will help correct the muscle tension and imbalance at the root of inefficient breathing, allowing you to become a far more efficient oxygen inhaler.

# **Preparation** and Mindset

The success of your 28-day somatic technique challenge depends largely upon thoughtful preparation. Here are half a dozen essential steps to take before starting the challenge:

**01**    Consult with Your Healthcare Provider

Before beginning the challenge, you should consult with your primary healthcare provider. This is especially important if you have any underlying health conditions or limitations. I recommend taking a copy of this book to show your doctor precisely what the challenge involves.

**02**    Set Clear Goals

Think realistically about the goals you want to achieve from the 28-day challenge. You should focus on retraining your nervous system rather than solely on outcomes. Somatic education aims to achieve proper bodily alignment and movement by releasing chronic muscle tension and improving awareness. Therefore, your goals should reflect this intention.

Instead of setting goals based on outcomes like weight loss or specific physical achievements, consider setting goals related to your somatic practice. For example:

- Goal: Increase awareness of habitual movement patterns and their associated tension.

- Goal: Improve the ability to perform pandiculations with focused attention and relaxation.

- Goal: Enhance proprioception and body awareness during daily activities.

- Goal: Reduce discomfort and pain associated with chronic muscular tension through somatic practice.

- Goal: Cultivate a mindful approach to movement and posture throughout the day.

By setting goals that prioritize the process of somatic reeducation, you can track your progress in developing healthier movement patterns and achieving lasting relief from chronic pain and tension.

**03** Purchase an Exercise Mat

Some of the exercises will be done lying on the floor. I recommend using an exercise mat for comfort and hygiene. Here is what to look for when choosing an exercise mat:

- **Thickness:** Choose a mat with adequate thickness to provide cushioning and support for lying on the floor comfortably.

- **Material:** Opt for a mat made of high-quality, nontoxic, durable, and easy-to-clean material.

- **Texture:** Select a mat with a nonslip surface to prevent slipping during movements.

- **Size:** Ensure the mat is large enough to accommodate your body comfortably and provides ample space for movement.

**04** Find a Sturdy Chair

Some of your exercises will be done while sitting in a chair. You should use the same chair every time. Here are the requirements for a good exercise chair:

- Sturdy base

- Not overly padded

- Backrest

- Armrests

**05** Create a Dedicated Space

Find a quiet and comfortable space in your home to practice the somatic technique without distractions. Your chair should have at least three feet of clear space around it to allow unrestricted movement. Ideally, a mirror should allow you to check your positioning and alignment when doing postural movements.

**06** Schedule Your Sessions

Block out dedicated time in your daily schedule for your somatic technique sessions. Whether you prefer to practice in the morning to energize your day or in the evening to unwind and relax, establishing a consistent practice time will help you prioritize your commitment to the challenge.

# 28-Day Somatic Exercise
## Challenge

# Your 28-Day Workout Plan

Once you develop the somatic exercise habit, you won't want to stop. These gentle movements are so effective at addressing the root cause of chronic pain that you'll wish you had known about them decades ago.

But building habits takes time. That's why I've presented the somatic exercises in this book as a 28-day challenge. Sticking to an organized plan for four weeks will ingrain somatics into your daily routine. You may struggle to stick with your new routine during the first week or two. But after that, it will become as natural a part of your day as brushing your teeth.

The 28-Day Challenge is organized around five key muscle areas:

**01**  Head and neck

**02**  Chest and arms

**03**  Abdominals and pelvic area

**04**  Legs and feet

**05**  Back

You will focus on these areas on consecutive days, performing 5 exercises from the 10 exercise selections I provide. On day six, you will restart with 5 more head and back exercises. You should perform the 5 exercises that you did not do last time. Continue this pattern for the entire 28 days.

Here is an overview of how the 28-day somatic workout plan will unfold for you …

| DAY 1 | DAY 2 | DAY 3 | DAY 4 | DAY 5 | DAY 6 | DAY 7 |
| --- | --- | --- | --- | --- | --- | --- |
| Head and Neck | Chest and Arms | Abdominals and Pelvic Area | Legs and Feet | Back | Head and Back | Chest and Arms |

| DAY 8 | DAY 9 | DAY 10 | DAY 11 | DAY 12 | DAY 13 | DAY 14 |
| --- | --- | --- | --- | --- | --- | --- |
| Abdominals and Pelvic Area | Legs and Feet | Back | Head and Neck | Chest and Arms | Abdominals and Pelvic Area | Back |

| DAY 15 | DAY 16 | DAY 17 | DAY 18 | DAY 19 | DAY 20 | DAY 21 |
| --- | --- | --- | --- | --- | --- | --- |
| Head and Neck | Chest and Arms | Abdominals and Pelvic Area | Legs and Feet | Back | Head and Neck | Chest and Arms |

| DAY 22 | DAY 23 | DAY 24 | DAY 25 | DAY 26 | DAY 27 | DAY 28 |
| --- | --- | --- | --- | --- | --- | --- |
| Abdominals and Pelvic Area | Legs and Feet | Back | Head and Neck | Chest and Arms | Abdominals and Pelvic Area | Legs and Feet |

# About the Exercises

Some of the exercises you are about to encounter may be familiar to you. Somatic movement is holistic rather than exclusive. As a result, it may incorporate poses from yoga, such as the cat-cow stretch and the bridge pose.

The key to maximizing the somatic benefits of each move is not the technical performance of the exercise, though this is important. Instead, it is the mindful awareness and attention to sensation that truly unlocks your therapeutic potential. You will notice that each exercise has two sections:

**01**  How to Do It

**02**  Somatics Guidance

Take your time to fully engage with the exercise to engage the brain and central nervous system. Follow each of the cues given, paying attention to how your body feels and focusing on the internal sensations that arise. Remember that somatic exercises are about physical movement and cultivating awareness of the mind-body connection.

By tuning into the subtle sensations, you can deepen your understanding of your body's patterns and promote greater relaxation and release of tension. Allow yourself to be fully present in each moment of the practice, honoring the process of self-discovery and healing that somatics offers.

# Head & Neck

Are you constantly dealing with neck strain? Do you get tension headaches throughout the day? Does your shoulder and neck area feel overly tight and constricted?

If you experience any of these things, the cause is likely the way you use your body throughout the day. You may have developed the habit of slumping in front of the TV or computer for hours on end. When this happens, your brain teaches your shoulder and neck muscles to remain tight and rigid all day, even at night.

This results in chronic tension and stiffness, leading to discomfort and pain. Tightness in neck muscles can also contribute to tension headaches, as the strained muscles can trigger pain that radiates to the head. But with targeted somatic exercises, you can break this cycle and find relief.

By releasing all the tension in your neck, you'll alleviate discomfort and reduce the frequency and intensity of tension headaches.

The nine exercises in this section will help to retrain your brain/ muscle connection. This will loosen up the neck muscles, releasing the tension built up over a lifetime and allowing you to rid yourself of the chronic neck pain you've been dealing with.

# Neck Rolls

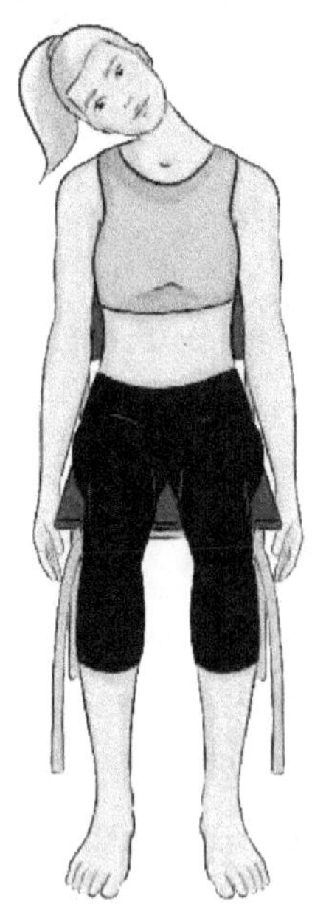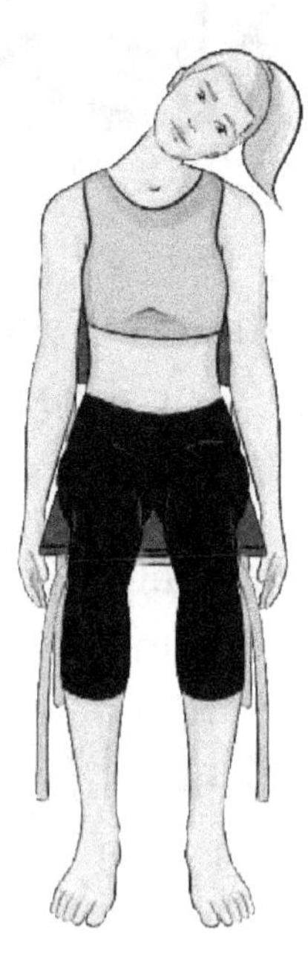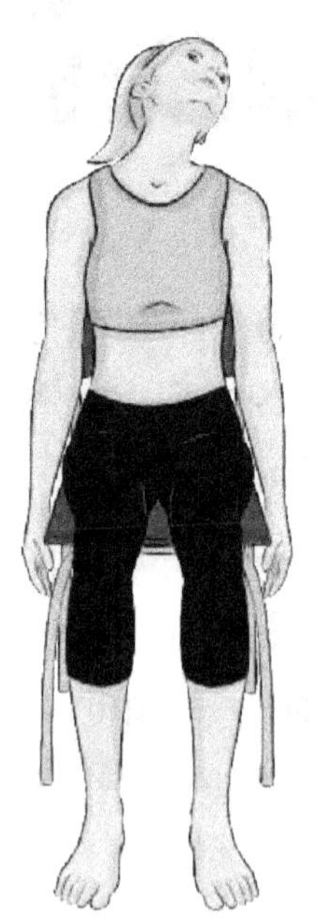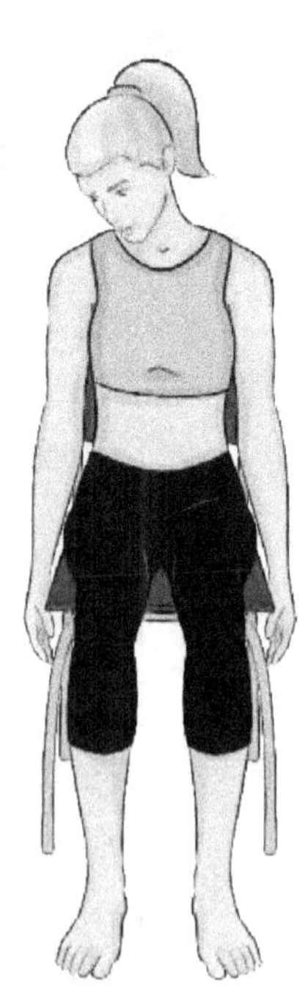

01 Sit or stand comfortably with your spine elongated and shoulders relaxed.

02 Slowly tilt your head to one side, bringing your ear toward your shoulder.

03 Slowly release your head back to the center, allowing the weight of your head to elongate the muscles along the side of your neck gently.

04 Gradually roll your head forward, bringing your chin toward your chest, and then slowly release it back. Continue the movement to the opposite side, again pandiculating back to the center.

05 Repeat this movement, alternating sides, for several repetitions, focusing on a slow release and controlled movement. Pay attention to the sensations along your neck and shoulders, breathing deeply and relaxing any areas of tension.

# Shoulder Shrugs

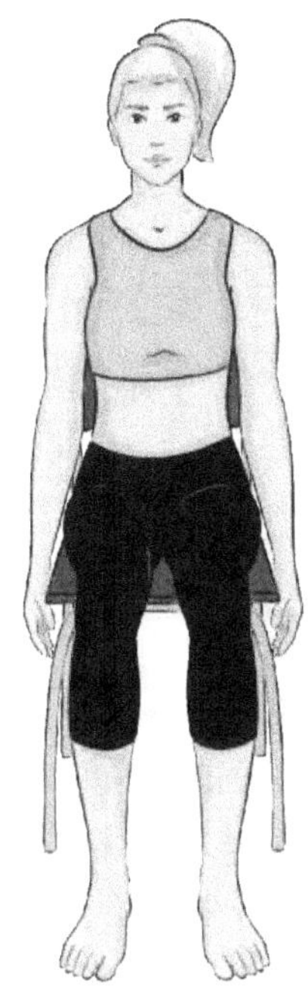 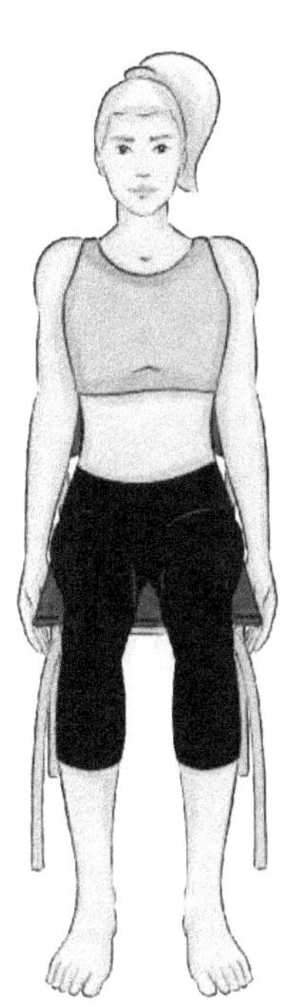

01 Begin in a comfortable seated or standing position with your arms relaxed by your sides.

02 Inhale deeply, lifting your shoulders toward your ears and engaging the muscles around your shoulders.

03 Exhale slowly, gradually releasing your shoulders back down to their neutral position, focusing on the feeling of tension releasing.

04 Repeat the shrugging motion for several repetitions, allowing each exhale to facilitate the slow release of tension.

05 Pay attention to the sensations in your neck and shoulders, noticing the engagement of your muscles as you lift your shoulders and the gradual release of tension as you lower them, ensuring each movement is smooth and controlled.

# Neck Stretch

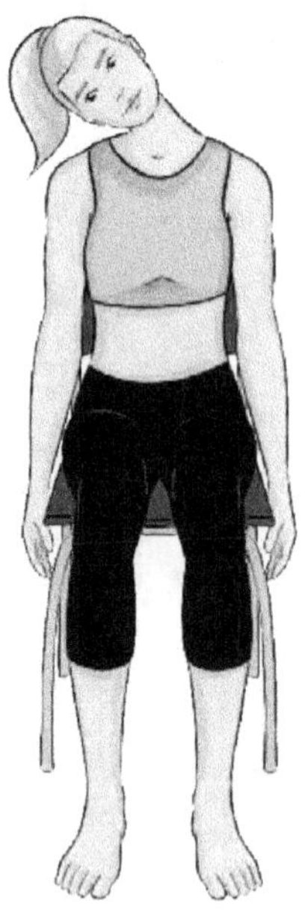 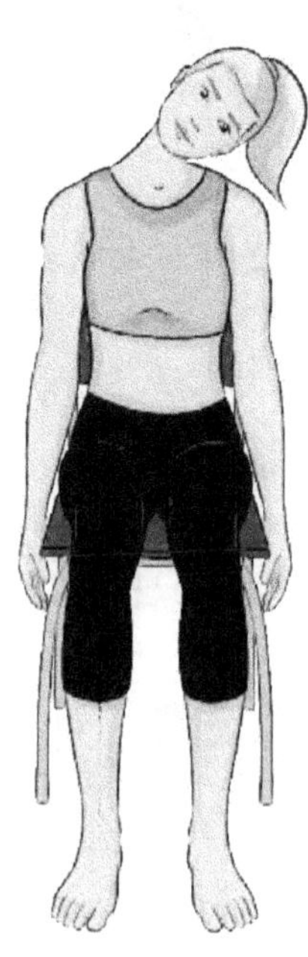 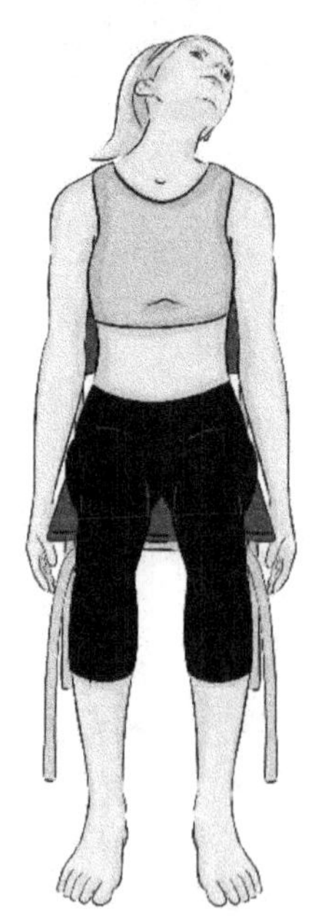 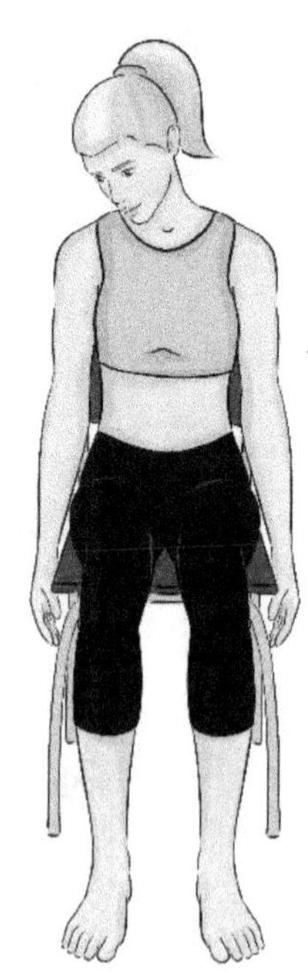

01 Sit or stand tall with your spine lengthened and your shoulders relaxed.

02 Gently tilt your head to one side, bringing your ear toward your shoulder.

03 Slowly release to bring your head back to center.

04 Switch sides, repeating the movement while maintaining deep breaths to aid in the slow release of tension. Pay attention to any differences in sensation between sides, maintaining a good posture throughout.

# Shoulder Circles

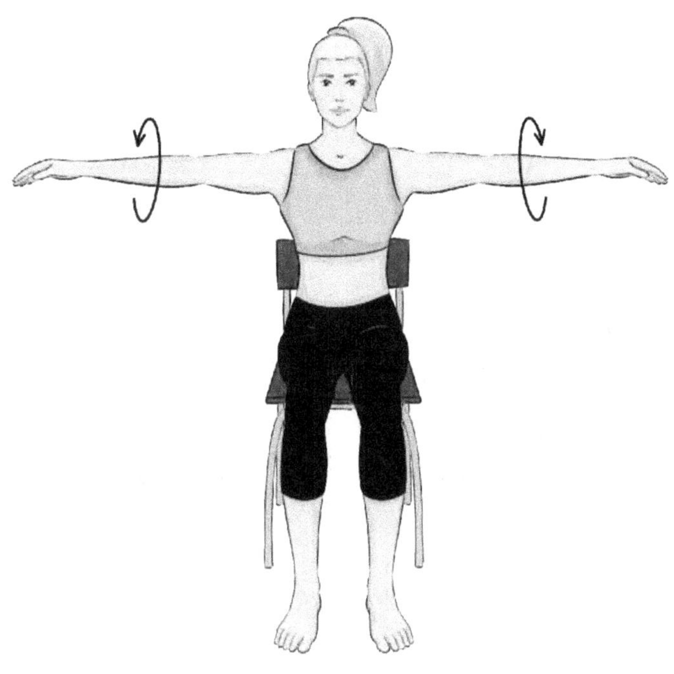

01 Begin in a comfortable standing position with your arms by your sides.

02 Slowly lift your shoulders toward your ears.

03 Slowly release them back down in a rolling motion.

04 Continue the circular motion for several repetitions, focusing on the slow release of tension in your shoulders and upper back.

05 Reverse the direction of the circles, rolling your shoulders forward and up, then back and down, again pandiculating.

06 Pay attention to the sensation of your muscles engaging and the range of motion in your shoulder joints as you roll your shoulders. Start with small circles and gradually increase the size, maintaining smooth and fluid movements throughout to facilitate the slow release of tension.

# Seated Levator Scapula

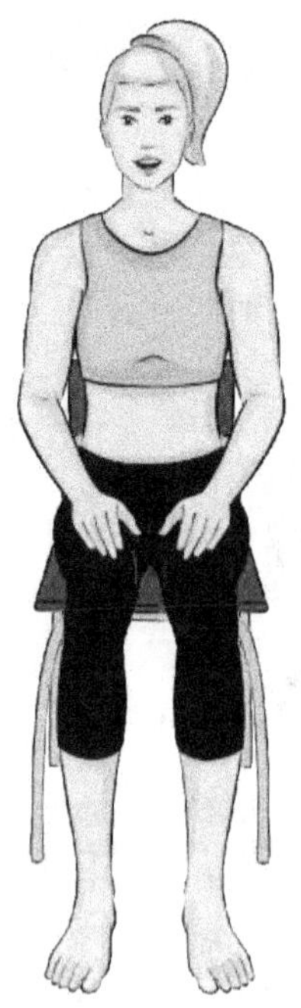 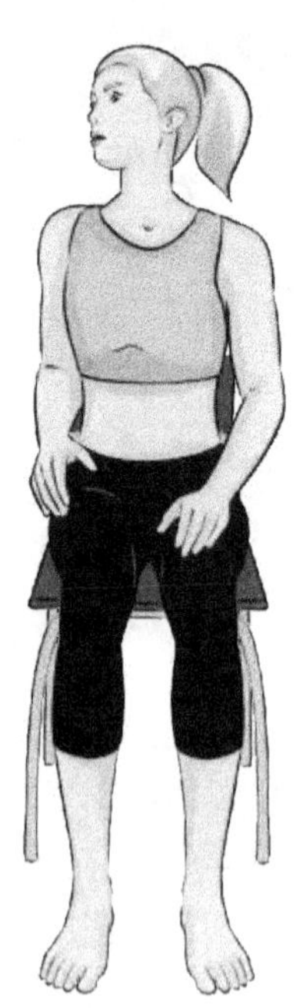

01 Sit comfortably with your feet flat on the floor and your hands resting on your thighs.

02 Turn your head to the right and then bend your right arm as you bring the right arm back and shoulder up, tilting your head back slightly.

03 Adjust your head to where you feel the tension in your scapula area.

04 Slowly release your shoulder and your head to bring the head back to center and place your hand back on your thigh.

05 Repeat on the other side.

# Shoulder Hunch and Release

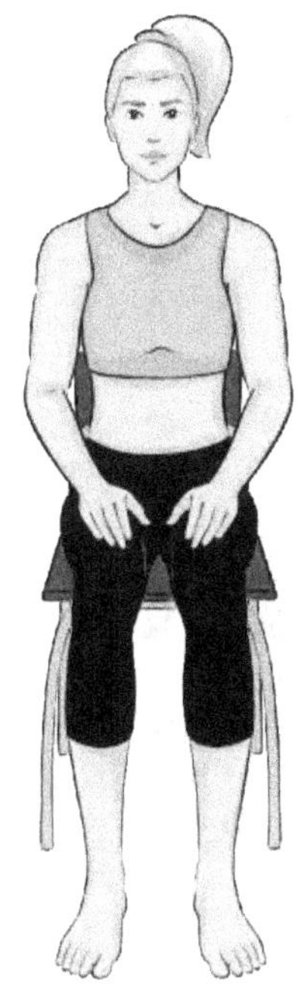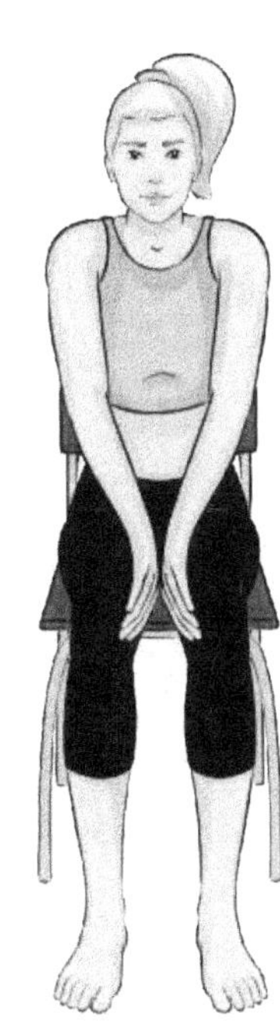

01 Sit comfortably with your feet flat on the floor and your hands resting on your thighs.

02 Roll your shoulders and arms forward and hunch forward, pressing your palms between your knees.

03 Slowly release, breathing naturally to come back to sitting normally.

04 Now, take your shoulders and arms backward to contract the muscles between the shoulder blades as you open the front of your body.

05 Slowly release back to a relaxed sitting position.

06 Repeat this backward and forward movement pattern to release tension between the chest and shoulder blades.

# Supine Spinal Extension

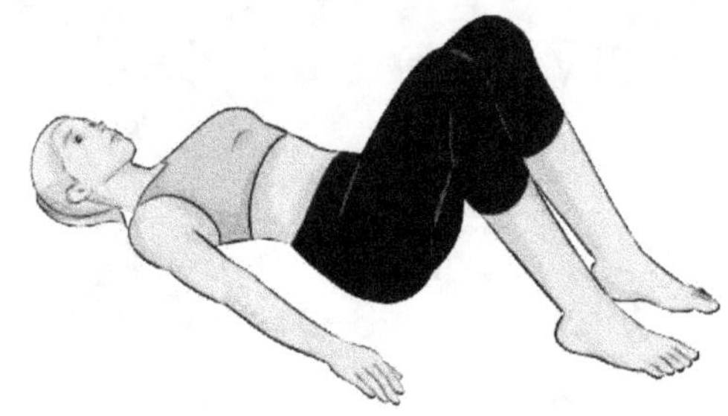

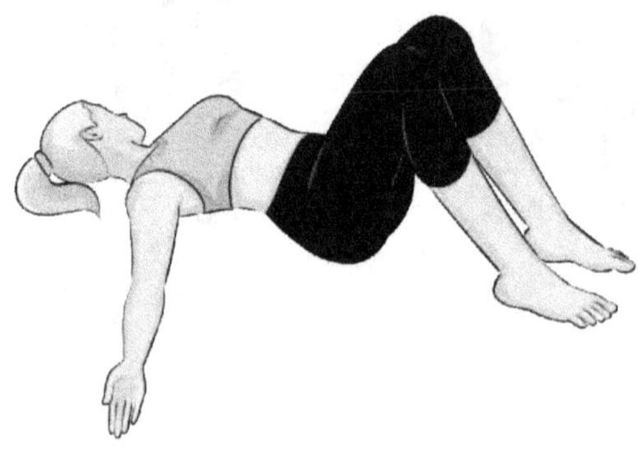

01 Lie on your back on the floor with your arms extended from your sides and feet hip-width apart.

02 Roll your face to the right, gently pressing the right side of your head into the floor.

03 Slowly release and let your face come back to center.

04 Roll your head to the right and press back again, this time also rolling your right arm outward so your right shoulder blade comes toward your left hip.

05 Slowly release and come back to center.

06 Now bend your knees and repeat, rolling your head to the right, tipping your head back and pressing it into the floor, and then rolling your arm outward to bring the shoulder blade closer to the spine. Allow your right hip to come up off the floor slightly.

07 Slowly release back to center.

# Neck Isometrics

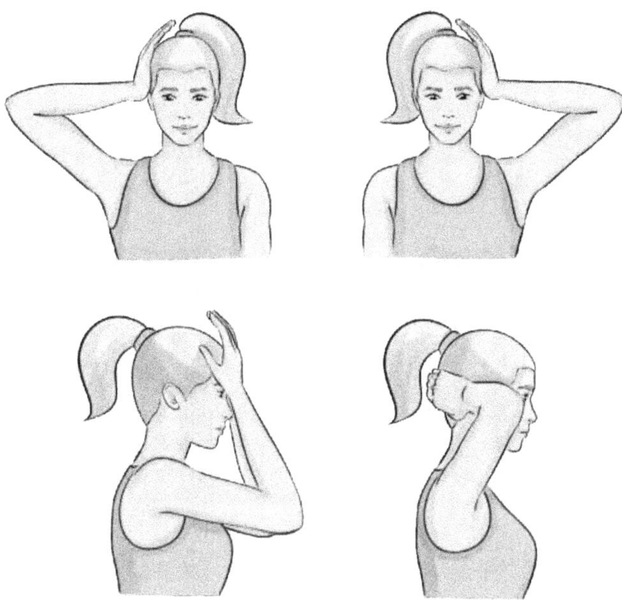

01 Sit or stand with your spine tall and your shoulders relaxed.

02 Place your hand on one side of your head and gently press your head against your hand, activating the muscles on the side of your neck.

03 Hold the contraction for 5 seconds, feeling the muscles working.

04 Return to center, engaging in a slow release motion.

05 Repeat the movement on the other side, gently pressing the hand to lengthen the opposite side of the neck.

06 Slowly release to return to center.

07 Now place your hands on your forehead and gently press your head backward, holding for 5 seconds.

08 Slowly release to return to center.

09 Finally, place your hands on the base of your skull and gently press forward to extend the muscles at the back of your neck, holding for 5 seconds.

10 Slowly release to return to center.

# Trunk-Shoulder Differentiation

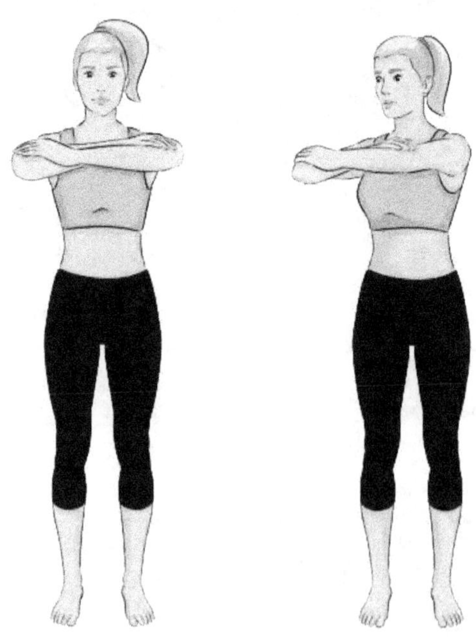

01 Stand with your feet shoulder-width apart and grasp your elbows at shoulder height.

02 Gently and slowly rotate your body to the left, back to center, and to the right side. Your entire upper body should move with you, including your head and neck. The spine, shoulder girdle, trunk, rib cage, and even your lower body should move slightly.

03 Lower your arms and relax.

04 Grasp your elbows again. This time, keep your head, trunk, and spine still as you move your shoulder girdle from side to side. Your arms, shoulders, and shoulder blades will be the only parts of your body that move.

05 Slowly lower your arms and relax.

06 Grasp your elbows again, and this time, keep your shoulder girdle still as you move your head, spine, rib cage, trunk, and neck from side to side.

07 Slowly lower your arms and relax.

# Chest & Arms

Chronic tension and discomfort in the chest and shoulder regions can significantly impede our quality of life. Add in the tingling sensations that may run down our arm into the fingertips, and you have a recipe for constant discomfort and frustration.

Whether it's due to poor posture, stress, or repetitive movements, these problems often stem from a condition known as sensory motor amnesia. This phenomenon occurs when the brain loses awareness and control over certain muscles, leading to chronic tension, restricted movement, and discomfort.

Incorporating somatic exercises into your daily routine can alleviate common chest and shoulder problems such as rounded shoulders, shoulder impingement, and upper crossed syndrome. The following somatic exercises tailored to the chest and arms will help release tension, improve posture, and reclaim freedom of movement.

# Chest Opener

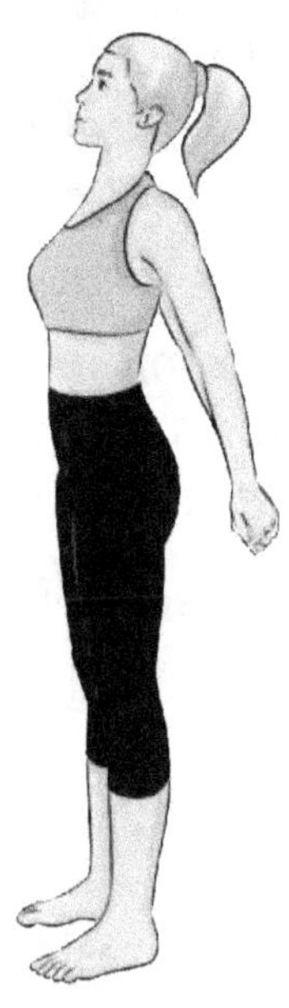

01 Stand tall with feet hip-width apart and your arms relaxed at your sides.

02 Interlace your fingers behind your back with your palms facing each other, feeling your shoulder blades draw together.

03 Slowly lift your arms away from your body, squeezing your shoulder blades together to open your chest.

04 Slowly release to return to center, ensuring your spine remains neutral and your shoulders stay relaxed throughout the movement.

# Wall Angels

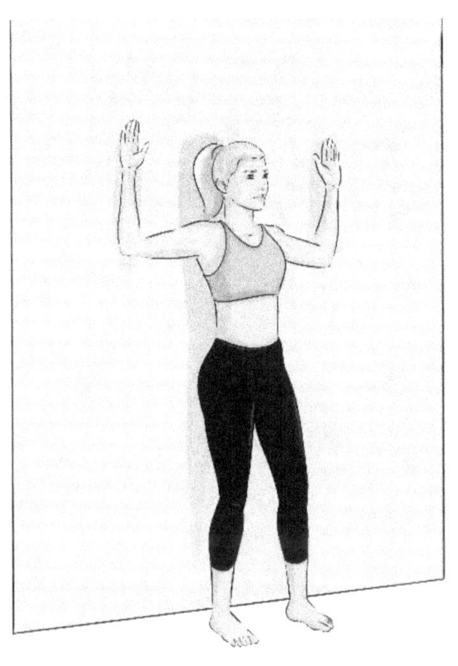 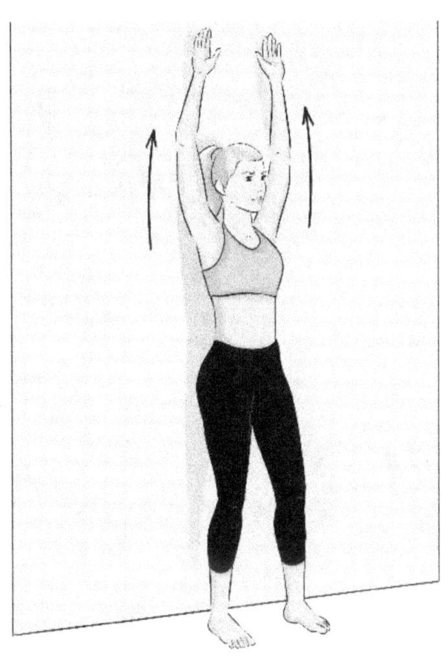

**Starting Position**

Begin by standing with your entire back pressed against a wall. Your feet should be about hip-width apart and positioned a few inches away from the wall.

This stance helps maintain a neutral spine.

**Pose 1**

Hold your arms up with a 90-degree angle at your elbows. Use the wall for guidance and resistance support.

**Pose 2**

Extend your arms upward. Drop back down to pose 1.

A variation is to extend upward and then bring your hands together in a prayer pose pointing to the sky. Then, drop back down to pose 1.

**Repeat for 10 reps.**

**Tip:**

If the pose is difficult for you or you're rehabilitating from an injury, prioritize form over range of motion. As your shoulder mobility improves, the movement may become easier.

As you gain strength and postural awareness, you can do this without the support of the wall.

# Chest Expansion

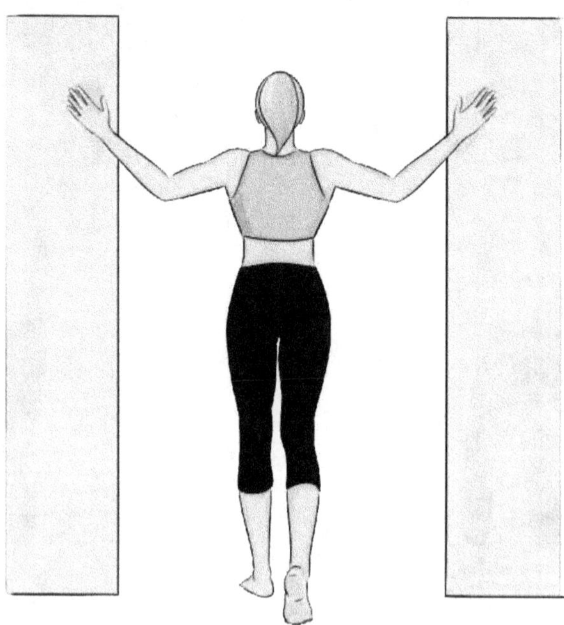

01 Stand in a doorway with feet hip-width apart, arms bent at 90-degree angles, and forearms resting against the doorframe, engaging in a pandiculation motion.

02 Lean forward slightly, allowing your chest to expand as you gently push against the doorframe.

03 As you lean into the doorway, deepen your breath and notice the sensation of your chest opening and expanding. If comfortable, gradually increase pressure but avoid any discomfort to facilitate the slow release.

04 Slowly release back to the starting position, taking about 5 seconds to do so. Maintain a neutral spine and relaxed shoulders throughout the movement.

# Spinal Arch and Flatten

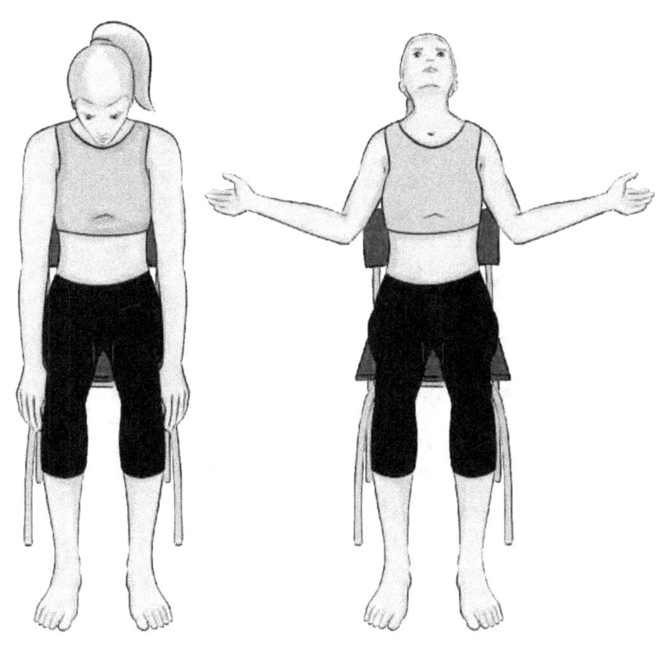

01  Sit comfortably with your feet flat on the floor and your arms at your sides.

02  Inhale as you roll your shoulders forward, lower your head, and curl your arms up to your shoulder level.

03  Slowly release to return to a neutral position.

04  Now extend your arms behind you as you inhale and arch gently by raising your head and chest. Extend your shoulders and elbows.

05  Slowly release to return to center.

# Seated Pectoral Muscles

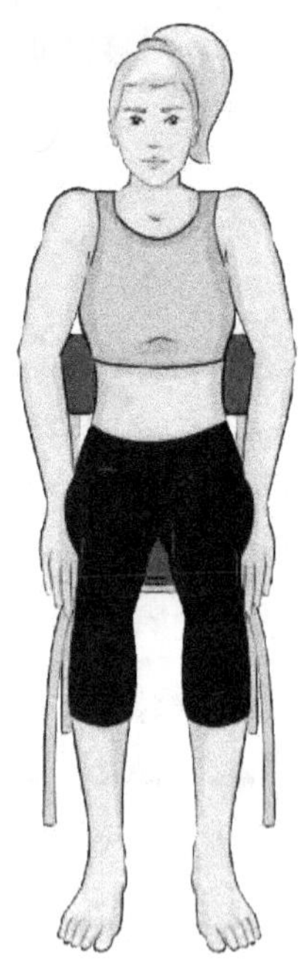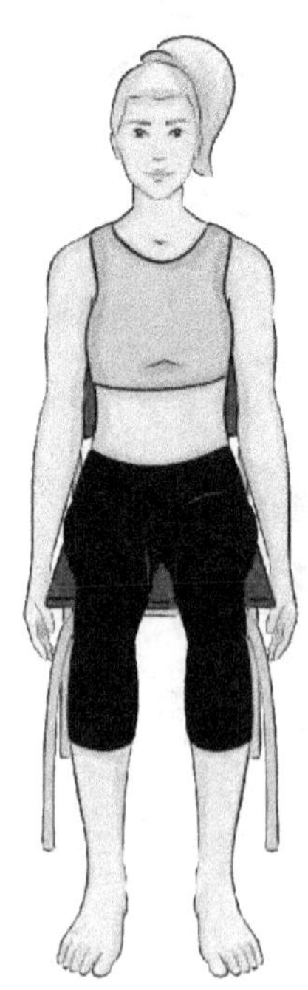

01 Sit comfortably with your feet flat on the floor, and arms at your sides.

02 Roll your arms and shoulders in, folding your belly in slightly at the same time. Bring your head forward slightly, too.

03 Slowly release to come back to center.

Note:

If your chair has armrests, place your arms on them while bringing your shoulders forward and your elbows up, contracting your belly and bringing your head forward. Then slowly release, leaving your arms on the armrests.

# Butterfly Hug

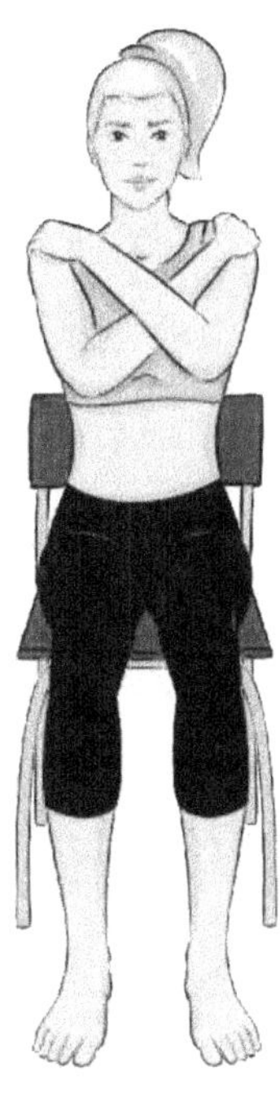

01 Sit or stand with a tall spine and relaxed shoulders.

02 Cross your arms over your chest, placing your hands on your shoulders with your fingertips touching your collarbone.

03 Inhale deeply, feeling a gentle expansion across your chest as you gently hug yourself.

04 Turn slightly to the right.

05 Slowly release to return to center as you exhale.

06 Repeat the movement, turning slightly to the left side.

07 Use your breath to guide the movement, inhaling as you open and exhaling as you close. Keep your spine tall and your shoulders relaxed throughout, allowing for fluid movement.

# Wrist Curls

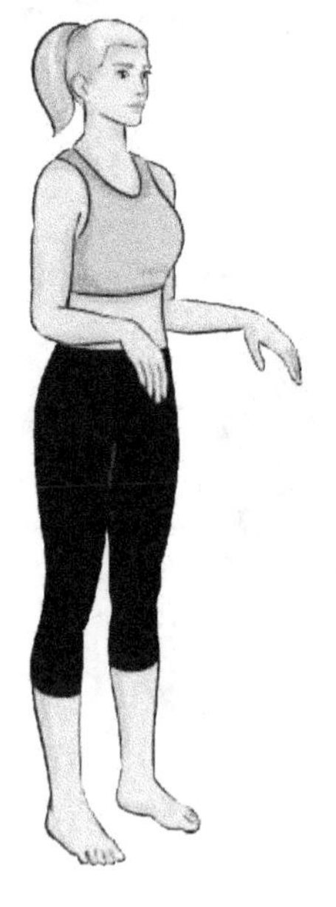 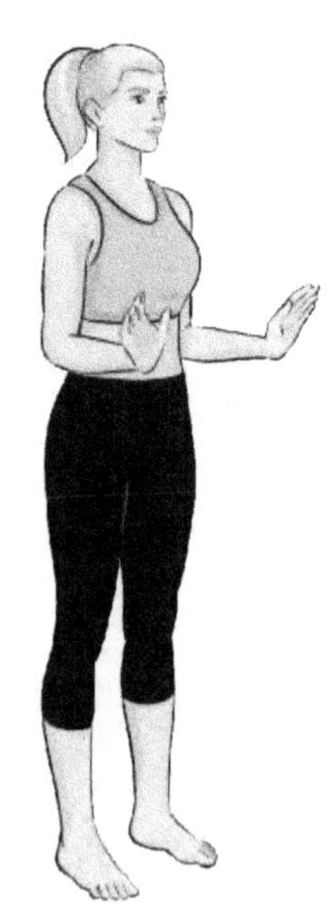

01 Stand or sit with a tall spine and relaxed shoulders.

02 Bend your elbows and extend your lower arms in front of you, palms facing down.

03 Lower your palms to the floor to contract through the wrists.

04 Slowly release, taking about 5 seconds to return to the center position.

05 Now, raise your fingertips toward the ceiling to contract in the opposite direction.

06 Slowly release, taking about 5 seconds to come back to center.

# Tricep Pandiculation

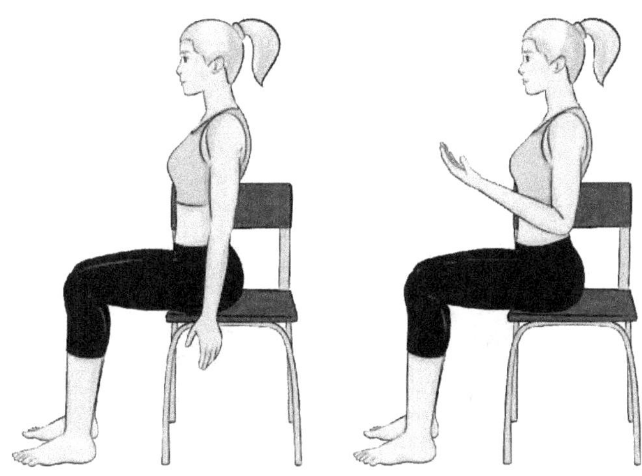

01  Sit comfortably with your feet flat on the floor and your arms at your sides, palms facing your thighs.

02  Flex your left elbow to bring the lower arm up to 90 degrees of elbow flexion.

03  Slowly, with control, release back to the starting position.

04  Repeat the process. This time on the release, stop a third of the way down and do a small recontraction.

05  Slowly release again, stopping again, this time two-thirds of the way down, and perform another small recontraction.

06  Slowly release back to the starting position.

07  Repeat on the other side.

# Arm Flexion and Extension

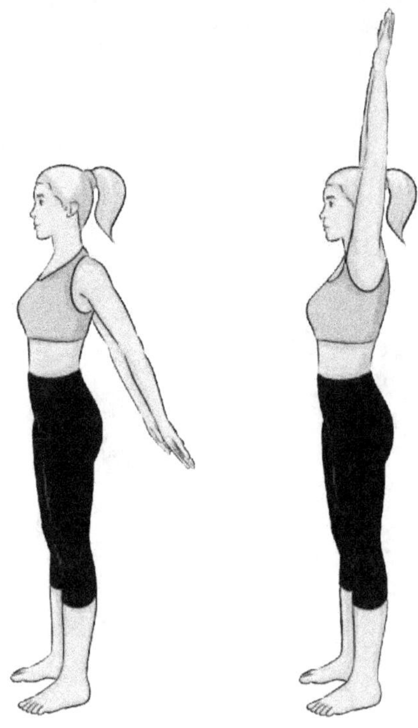

01 Stand with your feet hip-width apart and your arms relaxed at your sides.

02 Inhale deeply, slowly releasing both arms forward and up toward the ceiling, reaching as high as is comfortable.

03 Exhale slowly, gradually lowering your arms back down to your sides, maintaining a gentle release in the chest and shoulders. Imagine that you are melting into the floor as you bring your arms down.

04 Throughout the movement, keep your shoulders relaxed, your neck long, and use your breath to synchronize with the movement—inhaling as you raise your arms and exhaling as you very slowly bring them back down.

# Bicep Pandiculation

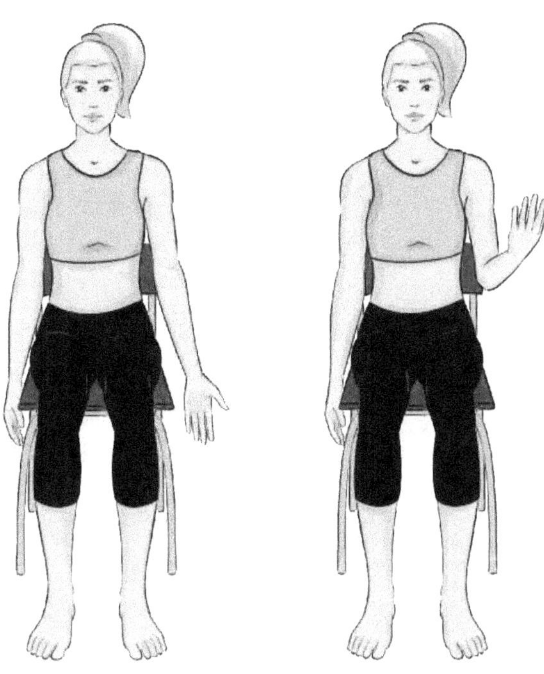

01 Sit with your feet flat on the floor and your arms at your sides with your palms facing forward.

02 Flex your left elbow to bring the lower arm up 90 degrees.

03 Slowly, with control, release back to the starting position.

04 Repeat the process. This time, when you release, stop a third of the way down and do a small recontraction.

05 Slowly release again, stopping again, this time two-thirds of the way down, and perform another small recontraction.

06 Slowly release back to the start position.

07 Repeat on the other side.

# Abdominals & Pelvic Area

Many people experience a lack of awareness and connection with their core muscles, leading to weak abdominals, poor posture, and pelvic floor dysfunction. These problems not only affect our physical well-being but also impact our overall quality of life.

Somatics offers a holistic approach to addressing these issues by reeducating the nervous system and restoring optimal movement patterns from the inside out.

By incorporating somatic exercises tailored to the abdominals and pelvic floor into your daily routine, you can alleviate common problems such as:

- Weak Abdominals

- Pelvic Floor Dysfunction

- Poor Posture

The ten following somatic exercises aim to awaken and strengthen the deep core muscles, including the abdominals, pelvic floor, lower back, and hips.

# Pelvic Tilt

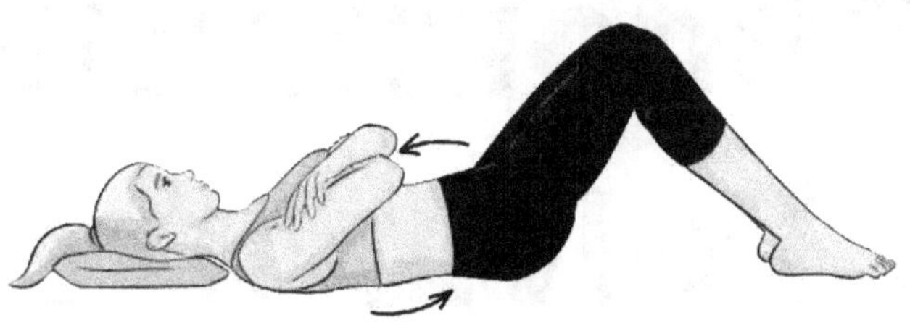

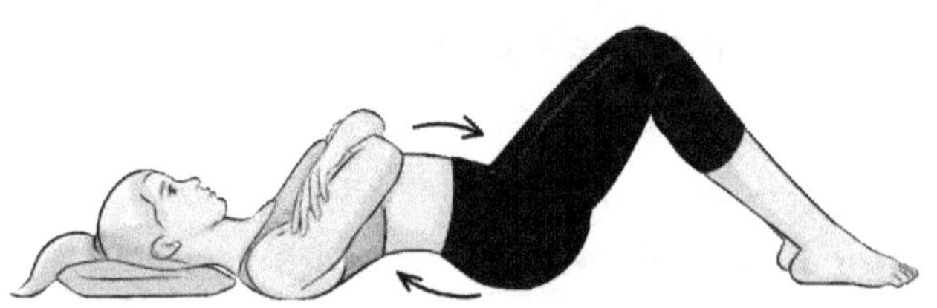

01 Lie on your back with your knees bent and your feet flat on the floor, hip-width apart.

02 Place your hands on your hips to guide the movement.

03 Inhale deeply and slowly tilt your pelvis back, gently pressing your lower back into the floor.

04 Exhale slowly, gradually returning to a neutral position, maintaining a slight arch in your lower back, pandiculating as you release.

05 Focus on the slow release and engagement of your lower abdominals and your pelvis's smooth, controlled movement. Throughout the exercise, keep your upper body relaxed and your breathing steady. Avoid tensing your neck or shoulders, allowing your pelvis to move with ease and grace.

# Abdominal Breathing

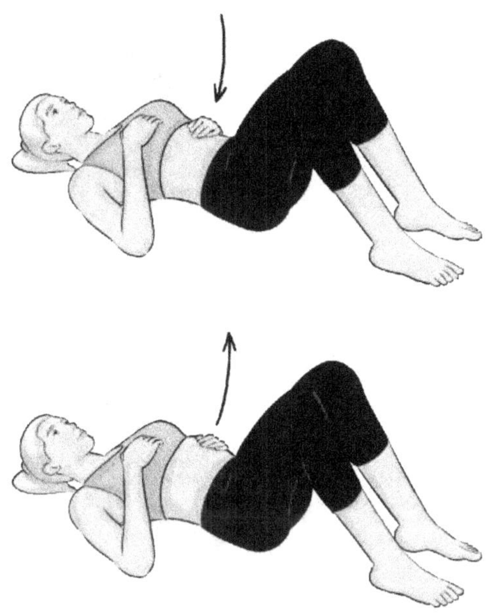

01 Lie on your back with your knees bent and your feet flat on the floor, hip-width apart.

02 Place one hand on your chest and the other on your abdomen.

03 Inhale deeply through your nose, slowly releasing as you allow your abdomen to rise and expand as you feel it filling.

04 Exhale fully through your mouth and very slowly release the tension through your abdomen, gradually drawing your navel toward your spine, feeling your abdomen contract as you engage your deep core muscles.

05 Throughout the movement, keep your chest relaxed, your shoulders soft, and allow your breath to guide the movement, creating a smooth and rhythmic pattern to relax and release tension. Imagine that you are melting into the floor as you release.

# Psoas Release

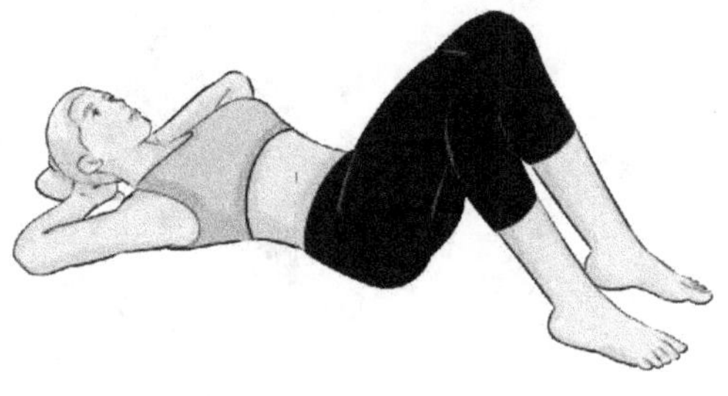

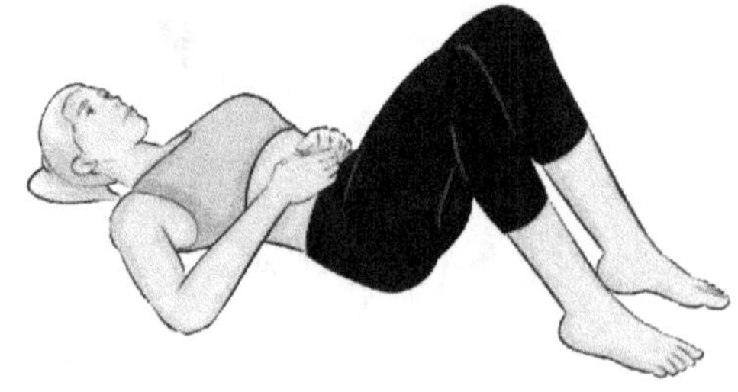

01 Lie on the floor on your back with your knees bent and arms by your sides, palms facing forward.

02 Take slow, deep breaths into your belly and exhale slowly.

03 Gently press your sacrum down into the floor, then very slowly release.

04 Repeat 2–3 times.

05 Keeping your lower back flat on the floor, bring your right hand up behind your head and allow the elbow to fall out to the side.

06 Inhale deeply, then slowly exhale, strongly flattening your lower back into the floor.

07 Lift your head off the floor to curl up slightly, simultaneously lifting your bent right leg off the floor, keeping your back flattened into the floor.

08 Very slowly release, maintaining full control to return your head and foot to the floor.

09 Relax and repeat three times.

10 Repeat on the other side.

# Pelvic Clock

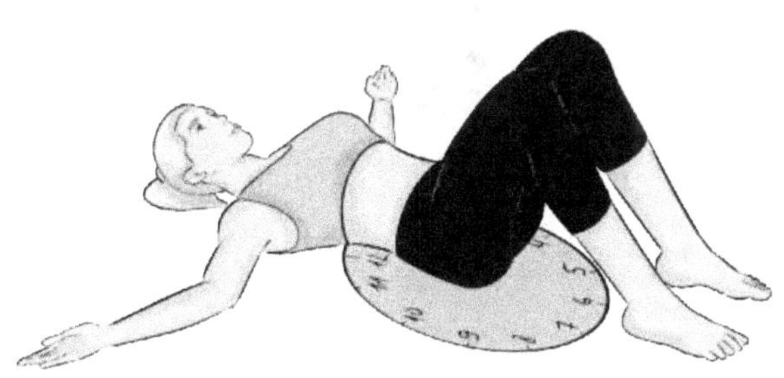

01  Lie on your back with your knees bent and your feet flat on the floor, hip-width apart.

02  Inhale deeply to prepare, then slowly tilt your pelvis back, gently pressing your lower back into the floor.

03  Slowly release as you return to a neutral position.

04  Now, tilt your pelvis forward, arching your lower back slightly away from the floor.

05  Slowly release, taking about 5 seconds to return to a neutral position.

06  Now, tilt your pelvis to the right, bringing your right hip toward your rib cage.

07  Inhale slowly for 5 seconds as you release to return to a neutral position.

08  Finally, tilt your pelvis to the left, bringing your left hip toward your rib cage.

09  Slowly release, focusing on the controlled movement of your pelvis, allowing your breath to guide the motion smoothly and effortlessly.

# Cat-Cow

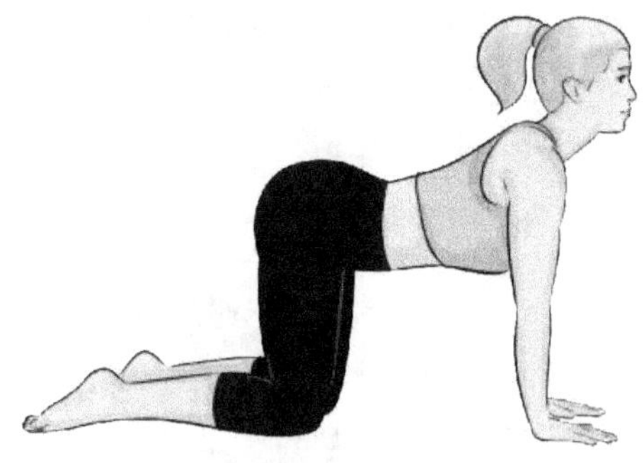

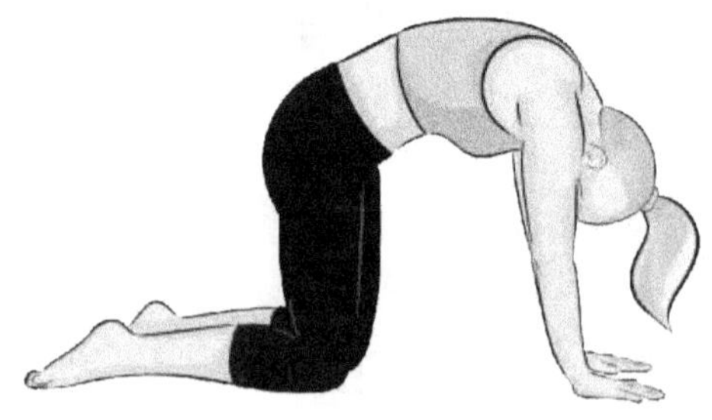

01 Start on your hands and knees with your wrists directly under your shoulders and your knees under your hips.

02 Inhale deeply as you arch your back, lifting your chest and tailbone toward the ceiling.

03 Slowly release, imagining your body melting into the floor.

04 Now, round your back, tuck your chin toward your chest, and press through your hands to lift your spine toward the ceiling.

05 Slowly release to return to a neutral position.

06 Continue moving between the Cat and Cow poses, with each breath flowing smoothly and rhythmically through the movements, focusing on your spine's slow release and controlled movement.

# Supine Leg Lift

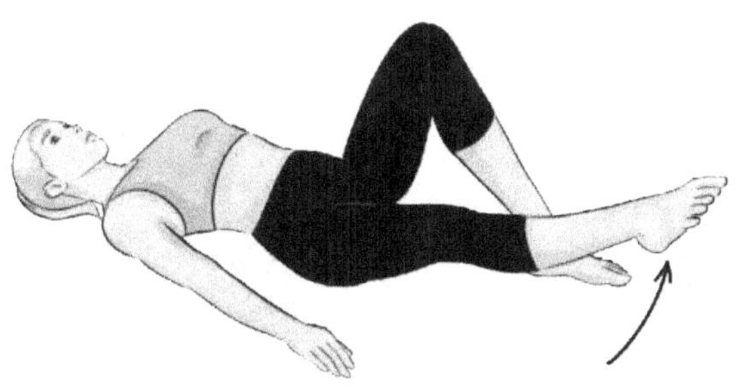

01 Lie on your back with your legs extended and your arms resting at your sides.

02 Slowly lift one leg off the floor, keeping it straight and in line with your hip. The leg should come up to approximately a 30-degree angle to the floor.

03 Slowly release it, taking about 5 seconds to lower the leg back to the floor.

04 Focus on the slow release and the sensation of your lower abdominals working to stabilize your pelvis. Throughout the exercise, keep your shoulders relaxed and your neck long, and allow your breath to guide the movement smoothly and effortlessly.

# Inward-Outward Legs

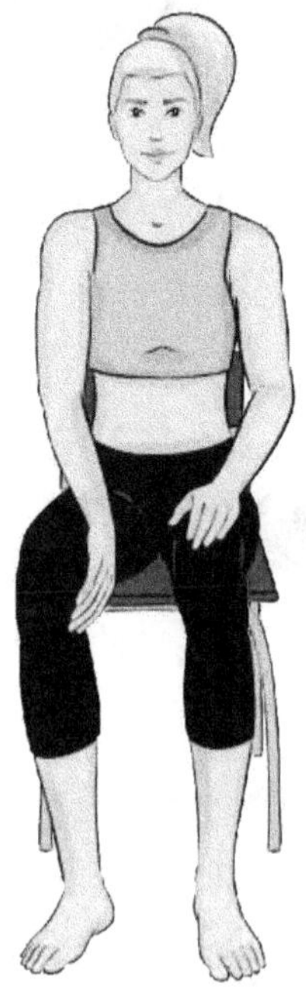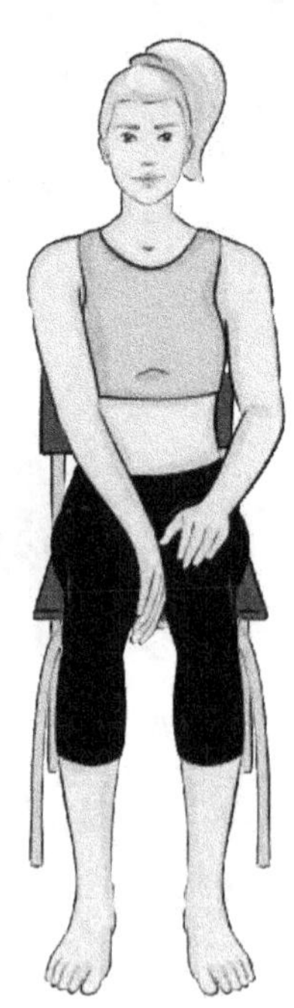

01  Sit comfortably with your hands on your thighs.

02  Breathe in, and then place your right hand on the inside of your right knee.

03  Gently press the knee inward to feel the knee moving into the hand.

04  Slowly release back to a neutral position.

05  Repeat two more times.

06  Now, bring your right hand to the outside of your knee and gently push the knee outward.

07  Slowly release back to a neutral position.

08  Repeat two more times.

09  Do the same on the other side.

# Bridge Pose

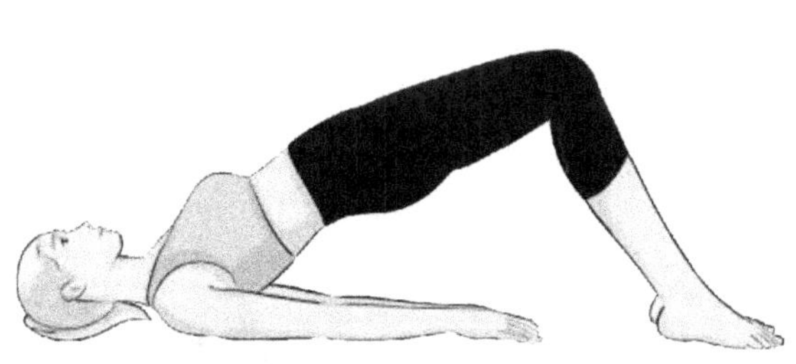

01 Lie on your back with your knees bent and your feet flat on the floor, hip-width apart. Place your arms at your sides with the palms facing down.

02 Inhale deeply to prepare, then slowly exhale for 5 seconds as you engage your abdominals, pressing into your feet and lifting your hips toward the ceiling.

03 Hold the position for 5 seconds, feeling a gentle release across the front of your hips and thighs.

04 Slowly release over 10 seconds, lowering your hips back down to the floor with control, pandiculating as you melt into the floor.

05 Repeat 5 times (or as many as you like until your muscles feel loose), focusing on the slow release and sensation of your muscles loosening. Throughout the exercise, keep your shoulders relaxed and your neck long, and allow your breath to guide the movement smoothly and effortlessly.

# Long Leg Psoas Release

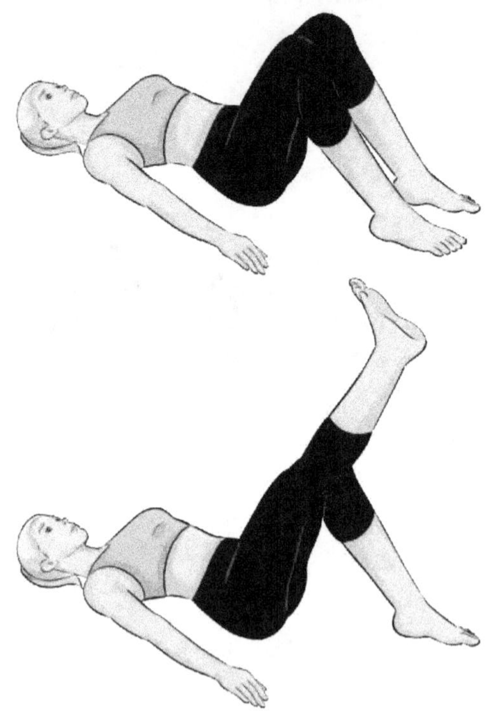

01 Lie on the floor on your back with your knees bent and your arms at your sides.

02 Curl your pelvis to engage your lower back extensors.

03 Slowly release to flatten out the pelvis.

04 Now lift your bent right knee and extend the leg so it is straight.

05 Very slowly release to return your leg to the floor, taking 5–10 seconds to do so.

06 Repeat on the other leg.

# Supine Spinal Twist

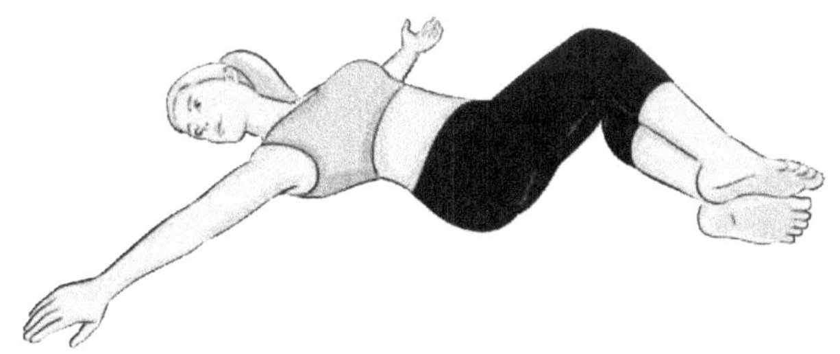

01 Lie on your back with your arms extended out to the sides at shoulder height and your knees bent.

02 Bring your legs to the left side, keeping the opposite shoulder on the floor.

03 Place your left hand on the right knee and gently press down. Keep your right arm extended on the floor.

04 Slowly release, taking about 10 seconds to return to center.

05 Repeat on the opposite side.

# Legs & Feet

Our lower extremities are the foundation of our movement. Yet, they often bear the brunt of daily stresses and strains. Many people experience a disconnection from their lower body, resulting in issues like tight hips, stiff knees, and achy feet.

By incorporating somatic exercises tailored to the legs and feet into your daily routine, you can alleviate common problems such as:

- Tight Hips: Prolonged periods of sitting and lack of movement can lead to tightness and restriction in the hip flexors, hamstrings, and glutes, resulting in discomfort and limited mobility.

- Stiff Knees: Lack of awareness and mobility in the knees can contribute to stiffness and discomfort, making activities such as walking and climbing stairs challenging and uncomfortable.

- Achy Feet: Standing for long periods, wearing improper footwear, and neglecting foot care can lead to foot pain, plantar fasciitis, and other issues that affect our ability to move comfortably.

The 10 exercises to follow will help you re-establish your brain's connection with your legs and feet.

# Tibia Toe Raises

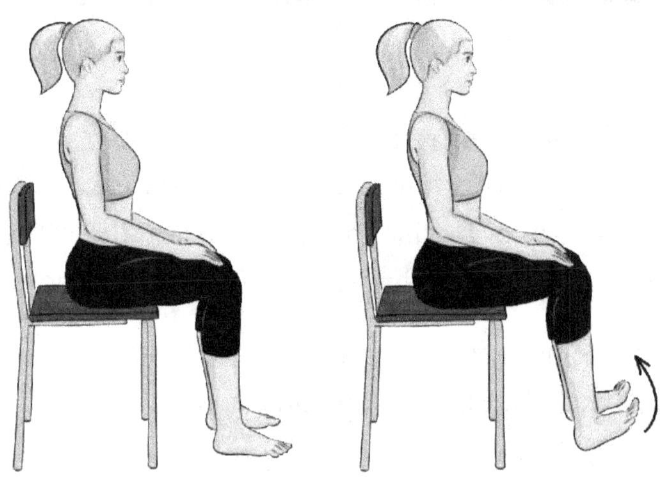

01  Sit on a chair with your feet flat on the floor and your hands on your thighs.

02  Raise your toes off the ground, keeping your heels firmly planted.

03  Hold the raised position for a few seconds, feeling the contraction in the arches of your feet.

04  Slowly release over 5 seconds to return your toes to the floor.

# Thigh and Hamstring De-escalation

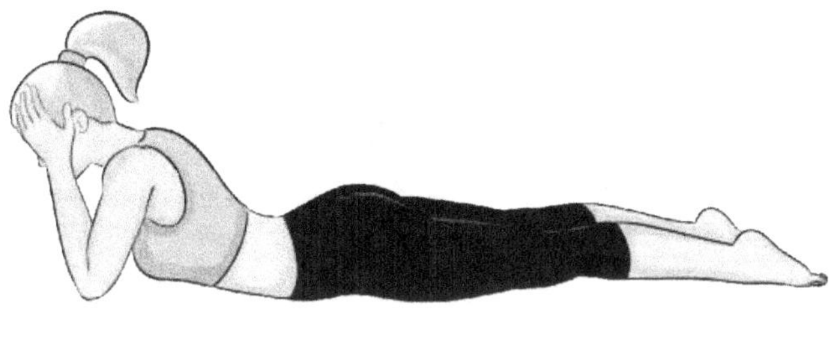

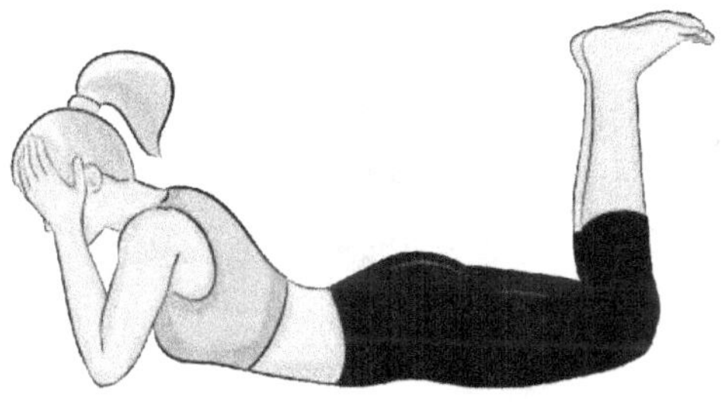

01 Lie on your front with your hands holding the sides of your head and your elbows on the floor. Bend your knees to lift your lower legs.

02 Place the right foot's upper part against your left foot's heel.

03 Push the two feet against each other. This will activate the right hamstring and the left thigh.

04 Allow the right foot to dominate as it slowly pushes the left foot to the ground.

05 Now allow the left foot to dominate as it gently presses the right foot back up.

06 Focus on the alternate relaxation and activation of the thighs and hamstrings.

# Side Bend

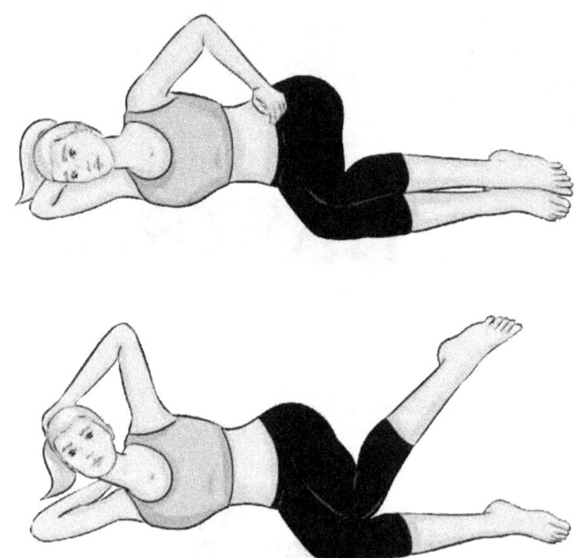

01 Lie on your back with your legs outstretched and your arms by your sides.

02. Roll over onto your right side and rest your head comfortably on your arm. Bring your knees up to your waist just as if sitting in a chair.

03 Place your upper hand between your ribs and hip bone, feeling the ribs with your fingers.

04 With your knees together, lift your top foot. This will rotate the top hip upward and inward. You should feel a contraction under your fingers.

05 Slowly bring your foot down and relax.

06 Repeat the movement.

07 Gently lift your head a couple of inches. You will once again feel a contraction of the ribs under your fingers.

08 Now, inhale before bringing your left arm over your head to grab the right side of your head. Exhale as you lift both your head and top foot, keeping your knees together. You will feel your ribs contract as the waist tightens.

09 Inhale as you slowly release to bring your head and foot back to the floor.

# Foot Pandiculation

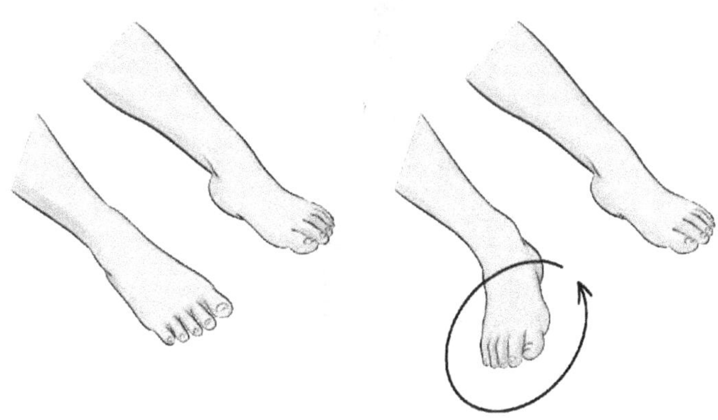

01 Sit on the floor with your legs outstretched and hip-width apart.

02 Place both hands under your right knee for support.

03 Flex the right foot toward you.

04 Now, very slowly lengthen the foot, and completely relax it.

05 Repeat two or three times, ensuring a smooth, gentle movement.

06 Now point the foot away from you to contract the calf muscle.

07 Slowly release it to return to a neutral position.

08 Repeat two or three times.

09 Now, turn your foot inward.

10 Slowly return it to a neutral position.

11 Finally, turn your foot outward.

12 Slowly return to a neutral position.

# Standing Forward Fold

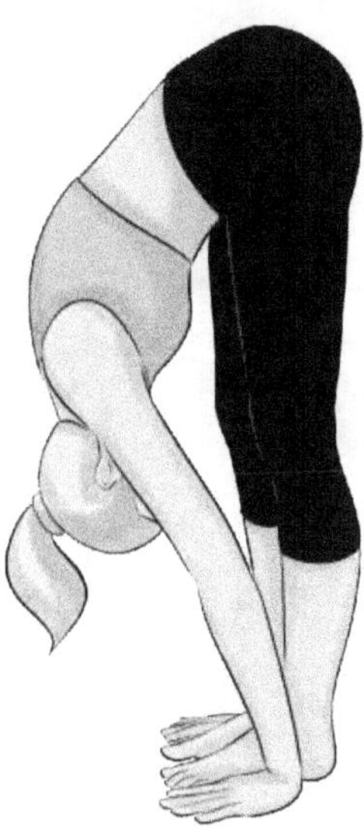

01 Stand tall with your feet hip-width apart and your arms resting at your sides.

02 Inhale to lengthen your spine, then exhale for 5 seconds as you hinge at your hips and fold forward, reaching toward the floor. Bend your knees slightly as you reach down.

03 Slowly release over 10 seconds as you inhale, gradually rolling back up to standing, stacking one vertebra on top of the other, pandiculating as you rise. Throughout the exercise, keep your shoulders relaxed, your neck long, and allow your breath to guide the movement smoothly and effortlessly.

# Washrag

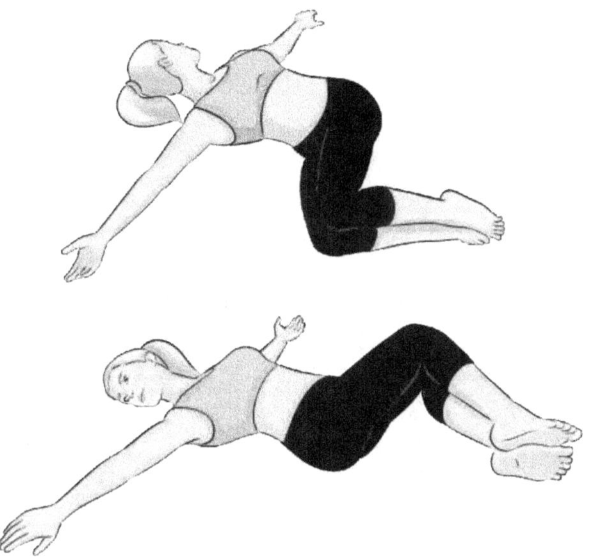

01 Lie on your back with your knees up and your feet planted near your hips. Bring your arms directly out from your shoulders into a "T" formation, keeping your elbows loose.

02 Imagine that your arms are rolling pins; turn one palm up and the other palm down. Allow your head to turn toward the upturned palm.

03 Alternate between palms, allowing your palm, head, and shoulder to roll further each time. You will be wringing out your shoulder like a washrag.

04 Stop with your head facing the upturned arm.

05 Allow your legs to gently drop in the opposite direction from your head. Roll on the outsides of your feet as your knees drop over.

06 Inhale as you come back to a neutral position.

07 Drop your knees to the other side as you continue rolling your arms and your head. Only go as far as is comfortable for you. Remember, this is not a stretching exercise!

08 Continue this slow, gentle movement several times. This will wring out the center of your body like a washrag.

# Seated Ankle Flexion

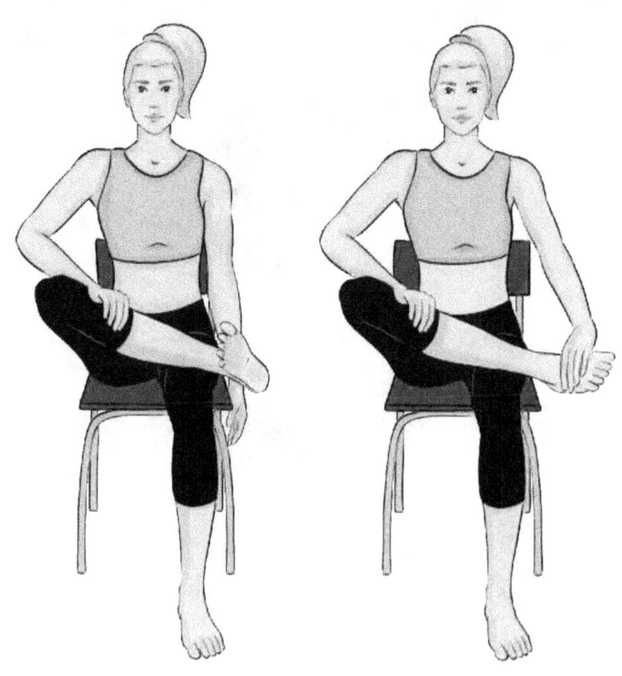

01 Sit on the edge of a chair and cross one leg over the other.

02 Place a hand on the top of the raised foot.

03 Now gently push against the foot away from you.

04 Slowly release to come back to a neutral position.

05 Place your hand on the underside of your foot and press the foot into the hand.

06 Very slowly ease off to return to a neutral position.

# Iliotibial (IT) Band Relief

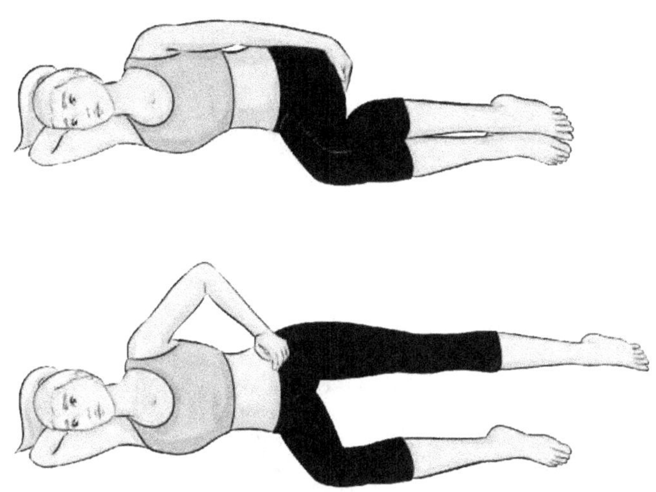

01 Lie on your side. If you have pain on the side of your legs, make sure the painful side is upward. Bend your knees and cushion your head with your hand.

02 Extend your top leg to the floor, keeping the bottom leg bent.

03 Flex the top foot, lifting it about four inches from the floor.

04 Place your top hand on the outside of your thigh and feel that your thigh and IT band are contracting.

05 Very slowly lower your leg to the floor. Once it makes contact, completely relax the leg.

06 Now lift the foot again, contracting the thigh. This time, you will also slowly pull your hip up toward your armpit using the muscles in your waist.

07 Slowly release to lower the leg to the floor again.

08 Now extend your arm up over your head and lift your leg, again drawing your hip toward your armpit.

09 Bring your extend up toward the ceiling and down toward your extended leg.

10 Slowly release back to a neutral position and relax completely.

# The Flower

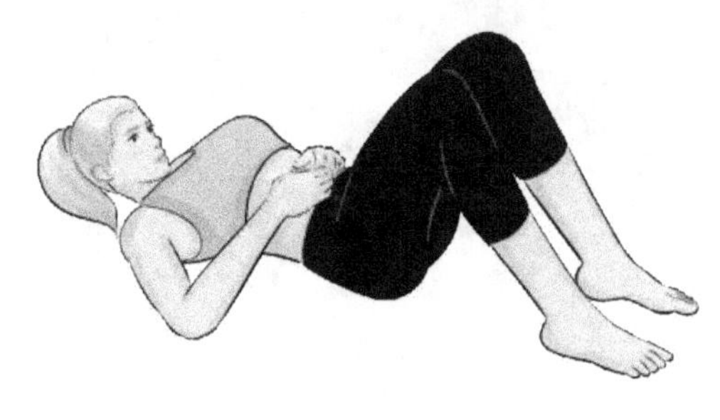

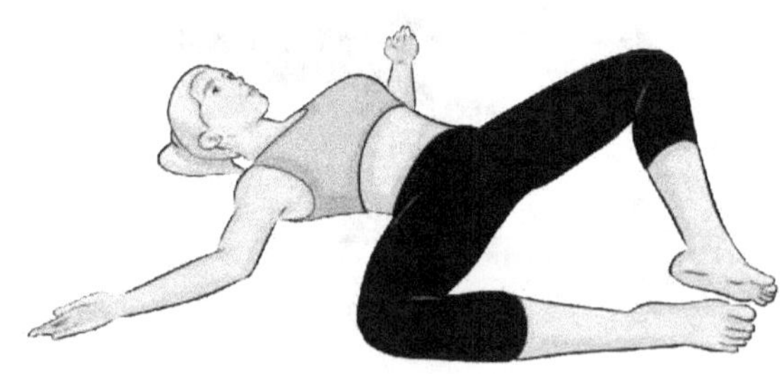

01  Lie on the floor on your back with your knees up and your feet planted on the floor.

02  Extend your arms at 45-degree angles to your body with your palms up.

03  Inhale and slowly roll both hands, arms, and shoulders inward toward your thighs. This will tighten your chest and contract your belly.

04  Inhale as you slowly roll back so your palms are again facing up.

05  Repeat the inward roll, this time allowing your head to arch back and your chin to extend toward the ceiling.

06  Inhale and slowly release to a neutral position.

07  Now, let your knees slowly drop outward until the heels of your feet face each other.

08  Exhale as you slowly come back to a neutral position.

# Seated Knee Circles

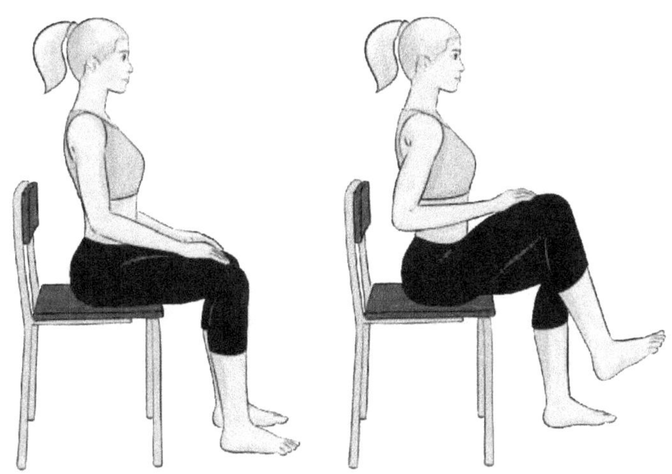

01 Sit comfortably on a chair with feet flat on the floor. Place your hands on your knees for support.

02 Rotate one knee in a circular motion, making one revolution.

03 Slowly release for 5 seconds as you reverse the direction and return to a neutral position.

04 Repeat the same movement with the opposite knee, focusing on your knees' slow release and controlled movement.

05 Perform 5 repetitions on each knee or as many as you need to feel the muscles around your knee loosening.

# Back

It's all too common for seniors to experience issues like chronic back pain, tight shoulders, and restricted mobility. These problems often stem from a combination of factors, including muscular imbalances, postural habits, and unresolved stress stored in the body.

Many common chest and shoulder problems, such as rounded shoulders, shoulder impingement, and upper crossed syndrome, are closely interconnected with back issues. By targeting the muscles of the back, including the erector spinae, latissimus dorsi, teres, trapezius, and rhomboids, somatic exercises can alleviate tension and strain in the chest and shoulders, leading to overall relief and improved posture.

# Back Lift

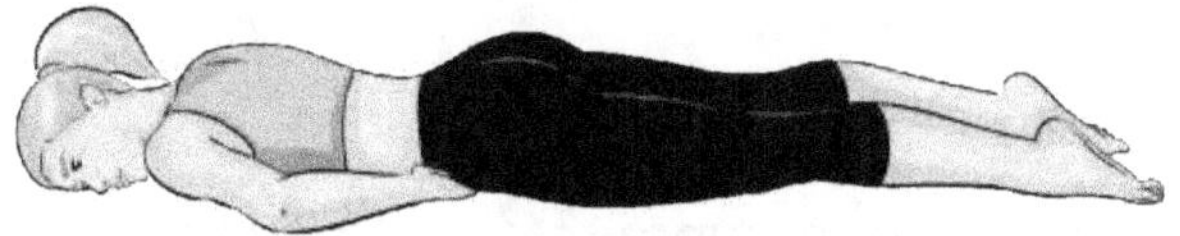

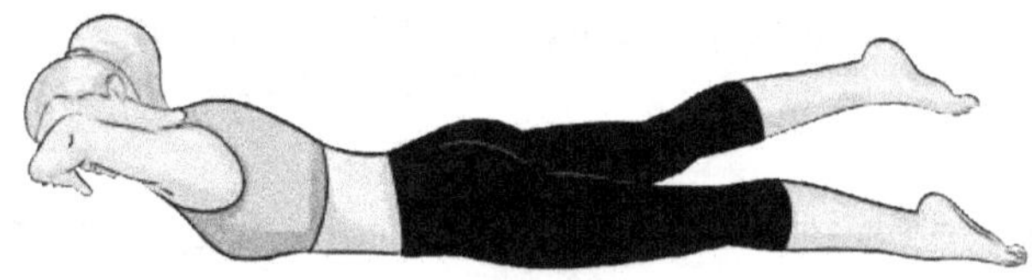

01 Lie on your stomach with your legs extended and your hands resting under your face.

02 Simultaneously lift your left leg and the front of your body. Bring your head and shoulders off the floor and look up.

03 Slowly release to lower to the starting position.

04 Completely relax as your body melts into the floor.

# Somatic Side Bend Variation

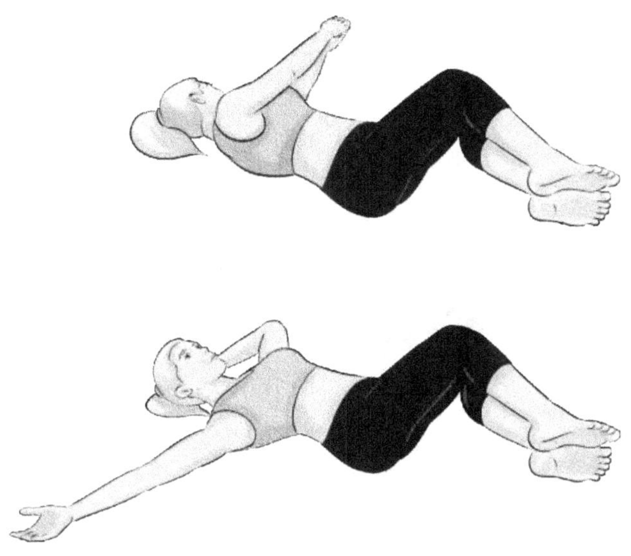

01 Lie on your side with your knees bent, both arms straight out, palms together.

02 Slowly bring the top arm up toward the ceiling and arc halfway down the other side or as far as is comfortable for you. Follow this arm movement with your eyes, neck, and head. Breathe through your belly as you do this.

03 Slowly bring the arm back to the neutral starting position.

04 Repeat two more times.

05 On the third repetition, stop when you reach the most comfortable point of the arm extension and put the opposite hand behind your head.

06 Now breathe in and, on the exhale, lift your head up toward the ceiling. This will contract the muscles around your ribs and waist.

07 Inhale and slowly bring your head down to completely relax.

# Sphinx

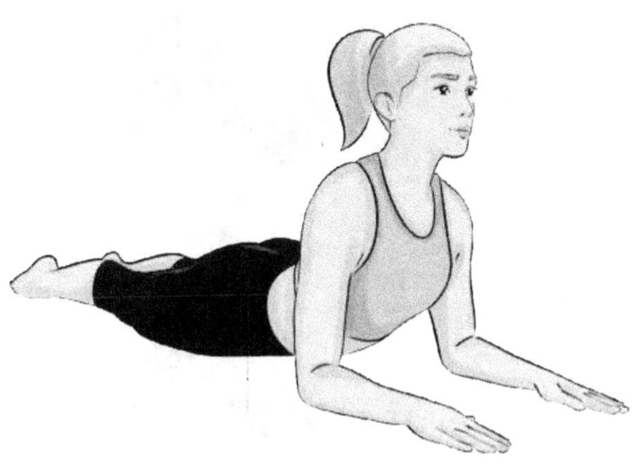

01  Lie on your stomach with your legs extended behind you and your elbows bent, placing your forearms on the ground in the sphinx position with your elbows under your shoulders and your fingers wide for support.

02  Press into your forearms and lift your chest, keeping your hips and legs on the floor.

03  Hold the pose for 5 seconds, feeling the gentle extension through your spine and front of your body.

04  Slowly release for 10 seconds as you lower back down to the ground. Throughout the movement, keep your gaze forward and your neck long, and allow your breath to guide the movement smoothly and effortlessly. Keep your shoulders relaxed and focus on maintaining a sense of stability and support in your core.

# Child's Pose with Reach

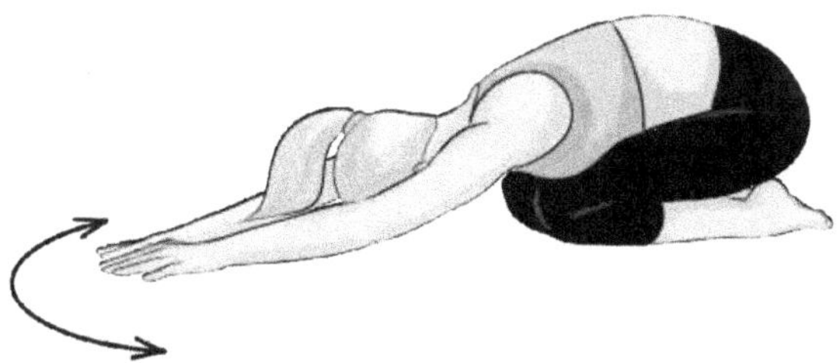

01 Start on your hands and knees with your wrists under your shoulders and your knees under your hips.

02 Lower your forehead toward the floor, extending your arms forward, and reach as far as you comfortably can, feeling your spine lengthen.

03 Lay your torso between your thighs.

04 Hold the position for 5 seconds, then slowly release it over 10 seconds to return to a neutral position.

05 Repeat the forward movement, this time turning slightly on the right side to engage the left side obliques.

06 Slowly return to center, then take another 10 seconds to return to a neutral position.

07 Repeat, this time turning slightly to the left side.

08 Slowly return to center, then take another 10 seconds to return to a neutral position.

09 Throughout the movement, keep your hips sinking toward your heels and your arms reaching forward, and allow your breath to guide the movement smoothly and effortlessly, focusing on maintaining a sense of ease and openness in your body while surrendering into the pose.

# Lower Back Pain Reliever

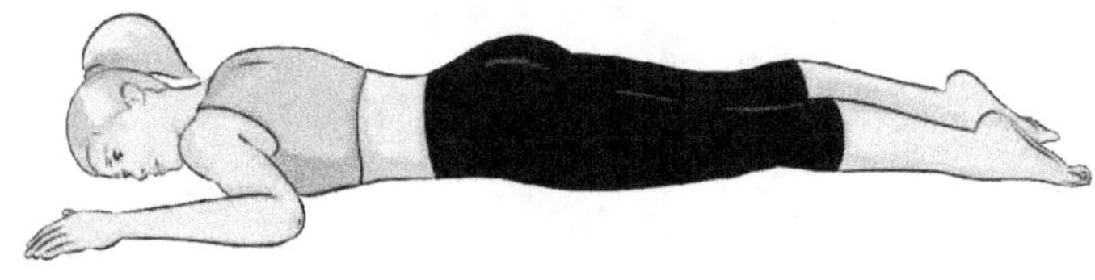

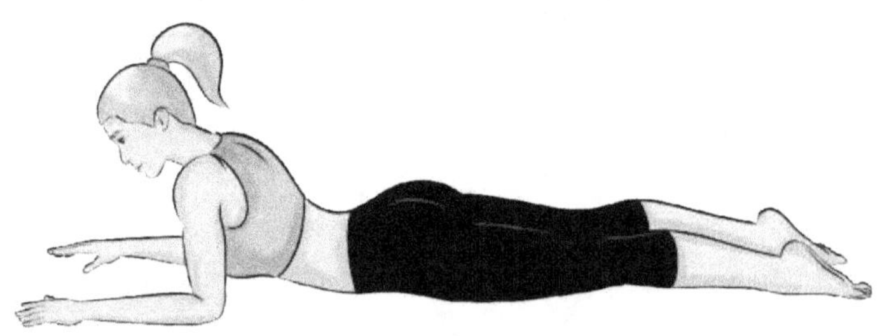

01   Lie on the floor on your stomach with your hands on either side of your head.

02   Inhale to soften your belly, then lift your head as far as you comfortably can.

03   Stop in the top position and feel the contraction of your erector spinae muscles that run alongside your spine.

04   Slowly release to soften and lengthen the back muscles as you return to the floor. Imagine your body melting into the floor.

05   Come up again, this time slowly lifting your head to the left side.

06   Slowly release to return to a neutral position.

07   Come up once more, lifting your head to the right side.

08   Slowly release to return to a neutral position.

# The Boomerang

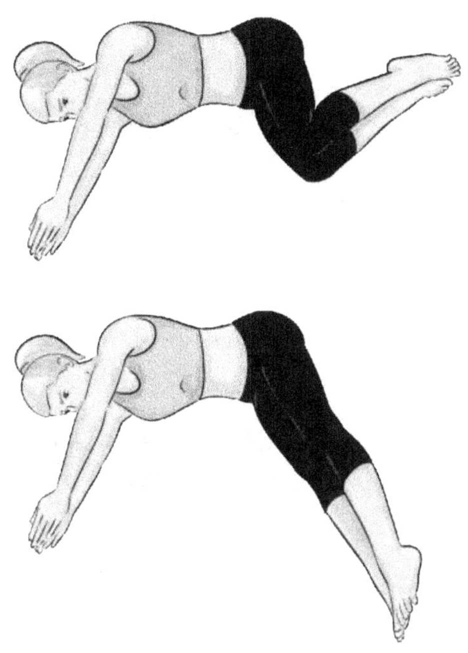

01 Lie on your side with your legs bent at around 45 degrees. Your arms should be stretched diagonally with the palms together.

02 Stretch both hands out in front and use your hands to support each other.

03 Inhale and relax your back as you extend your legs out comfortably.

04 As you release, round your back and allow your legs to curl back to its original position

05 That is it. A variation is to open up your arm and raise it in the air as you extend your legs out

06 Upon finishing 5 reps, let your body melt into the floor and rest here for a bit.

# Inversion/Eversion

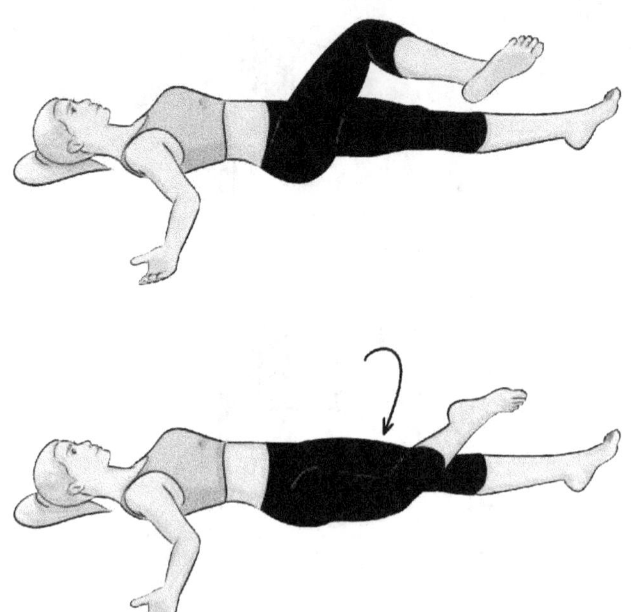

01  Lie on the floor on your back with your feet hip-width apart and your arms out to your sides.

02  Invert your right foot and scoop it toward the ceiling so it's facing your left foot, bending the knee outward. This will lift the opposite hip.

03  Slowly release back to the starting position.

04  Now, evert your foot so it looks away from your left foot, bringing the knee across the body.

05  Slowly release back to the starting position.

06  Repeat with the other leg.

# Superman Pose

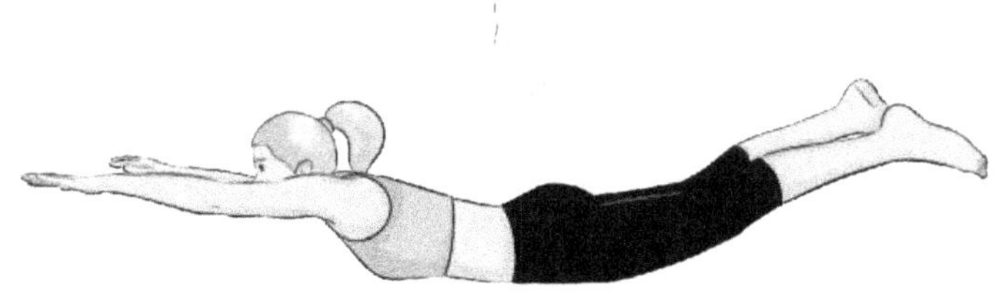

01 Lie on your stomach with your arms extended overhead and your legs straight behind you.

02 Lift your arms, chest, and legs off the ground, engaging your back muscles.

03 Hold the pose for 3 seconds, feeling the engagement of your erector spinae muscles.

04 Slowly release, taking up to 10 seconds to return to the starting position.

05 Throughout the exercise, keep your shoulders relaxed and your neck long and allow your breath to guide the movement smoothly and effortlessly, maintaining a sense of stability and control in your core and pelvis while avoiding any excessive arching or straining in your lower back.

# Twisted Curl

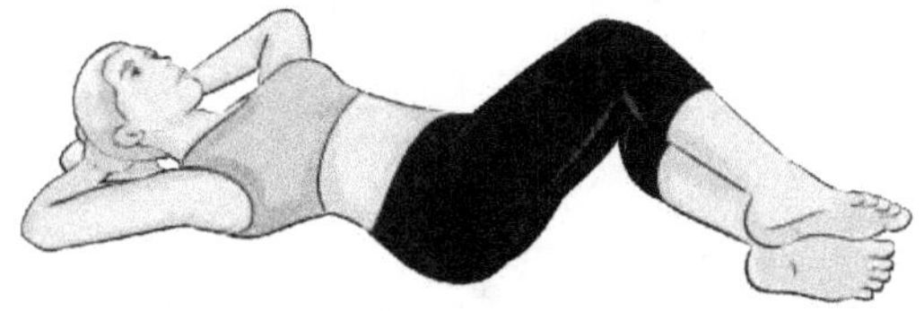

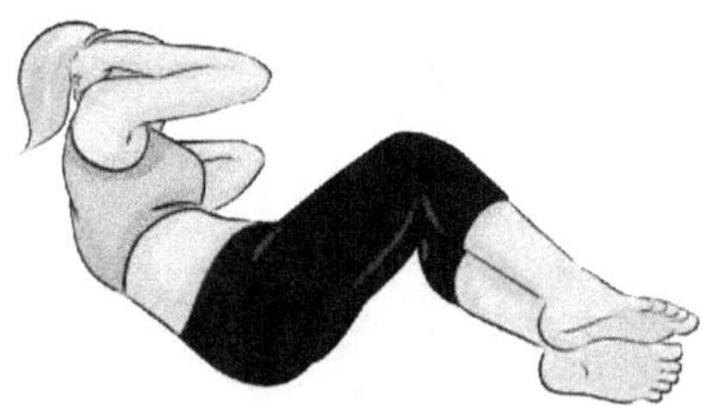

01 Lie on your side with your legs bent at around 45 degrees. Place both hands behind your head.

02 Turn your head, neck, and shoulder toward the ceiling to twist your upper body.

03 Curl forward with your shoulder, head, and arms as you bring both feet off the floor.

04 Slowly release to return to the starting position.

# The Road Ahead

As we conclude our 28-day somatic exercise journey, I want to thank you for the commitment, trust, and dedication you have shown. Somatics is a new and different type of treatment, and it's easy to dismiss it as just another fad. So, congratulations on being open-minded and willing to explore this innovative approach to wellness. Your commitment, trust, and dedication throughout this 28-day somatic exercise journey have been truly commendable.

This guide has provided you with a structured and motivating framework to incorporate somatics into your daily routine. The positive changes you've experienced so far are only the beginning.

Over the past 28 days, you have been able to retrain improper neural pathways that have been embedded in your system for decades. This has allowed your brain and your muscles to wake up from sensory motor amnesia. The results you have experienced are transformative ...

- Pain relief

- Relaxed muscles

- Increased mobility and flexibility

- Tension release

The 28-day program is just the start for you. Your commitment to the program has helped ingrain somatic exercise as part of your daily routine. I encourage you to continue this pattern.

The ten minutes you dedicate to somatic exercise every day will serve as a foundation for lifelong wellness and vitality. By continuing to prioritize somatic exercises in your daily routine, you're not only maintaining the progress you've made but also setting the stage for even greater improvements in the future.

Thank you for joining me on this somatic exercise adventure. Your dedication to self-care is truly commendable. May your journey toward a healthier, happier you continue to flourish. Remember, the benefits of these exercises extend far beyond physical fitness—they are a gift to your mind, body, and spirit.

I know that some of you will want to continue on to more advanced exercises, so before we say goodbye, let me direct you to our exclusive pelvic floor Kegels exercise guide at wallpilates.org as taught by Tim Sawyer, a leading physical therapist who worked with Dr. Anderson and Dr. Wise at the Stanford University Medical Center[1]. When you enter your email to download this free bonus, you'll also be notified of new Pilates books and workout routines we'll release in the future.

You can also scan the following QR code to receive your free bonus:

Wishing you continued success on your wellness journey.

Love, Luna

---

1    Wise, D. & Anderson, R. (2018). *A Headache in the Pelvis: The Wise-Anderson Protocol for Healing Pelvic Pain: The Definitive Edition. Harmony.*

# Thank You

My name is Luna, and it has been my pleasure to serve you. You could have picked from dozens of other books, but you took a chance and chose this one. So, thank you for investing in yourself and making it to the end!

Before we say goodbye, one question: If you enjoyed this book, would you consider leaving a review? A review is the easiest and best way to support the work of independent authors like me. Your feedback will help us continue writing the types of books that will help you and others in the journey to good health.

To leave a review directly, please go to this link:

https://www.amazon.com/review/create-review/?asin=B0D9NV69TN

You can also get your free bonuses here:

https://www.wallpilates.org/

*To your happiness and health*

*—Luna Light*

# Additional Resources

Use this URL from the National Pilates Certification Program to find a certified Pilates instructor:

https://nationalpilatescertificationprogram.org/NPCP/NPCP/Directory/CertifiedTeachersList.aspx

Find and add a certified yoga instructor search/association:

https://www.iayt.org/search/custom.asp?id=4160

# Disclosures

Some of the links provided in this book are affiliate links, which help you jump to the exact URL of the resource you're looking for at no additional cost to you.

www.ingramcontent.com/pod-product-compliance
Lightning Source LLC
Chambersburg PA
CBHW081223260726
48653CB00010BB/3767